EMT-BASIC

PRETEST® SELF-ASSESSMENT AND REVIEW

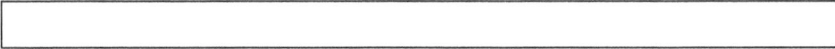

EMT-BASIC

PRETEST® SELF-ASSESSMENT AND REVIEW

Richard E.J. Westfal, M.D., F.A.C.E.P.
Associate Director
Department of Emergency Medicine
Saint Vincent's Hospital
New York, New York
Associate Professor
Department of Emergency Medicine
New York Medical College
Valhalla, New York

John Filangeri, E.M.T.-P.
Paramedic Program Director
Hudson Valley Hospital Center
Peekskill, New York

McGraw-Hill
Health Professions Division
PreTest® Series

New York   St. Louis   San Francisco   Auckland   Bogotá   Caracas   Lisbon   London   Madrid
Mexico City   Milan   Montreal   New Delhi   San Juan   Singapore   Sydney   Tokyo   Toronto

McGraw-Hill

A Division of The McGraw·Hill Companies

EMT-Basic: PreTest® Self-Assessment and Review

Copyright ©1998 by The McGraw-Hill Companies, Inc. All rights reserved. Printed in the United States of America. Except as permitted under the Copyright Act of 1976, no part of this publication may be reproduced or distributed in any form or by any means, or stored in a data base or retrieval system, without the prior written permission of the publisher.

1 2 3 4 5 6 7 8 9 0   DOCDOC   9 9 8 7

ISBN 0-07-052493-9

The editors were John Dolan and Peter McCurdy.
The production supervisor was Helene G. Landers.
R.R. Donnelley & Sons was printer and binder.
This book was set in Times Roman by V&M Graphics.

CONTENTS

PREFACE

Emergency Medical Technician-Basic: PreTest® *Self-Assessment and Review* has been designed to prepare entry level and refresher emergency medical technician-basic students for upcoming National Registry, regional, state, and city examinations. Additionally, this book provides information to assist EMT-Basic instructors, course coordinators, and medical directors in assessing the progress of their students.

In 1994 the United States Department of Transportation instituted a new curriculum for the training of emergency medical technicians. The title EMT-A (Ambulance) for the entry level was changed to EMT-B (Basic). All emergency medical technicians must pass a written qualifying examination in order to be certified or licensed to practice. In some cases these examinations are administered by individual states. The National Registry of Emergency Medical Technicians also administers examinations that are recognized by some of the states. Many emergency medical technicians must also take a state recertifying examination at periods ranging from two to five years. Most states have followed the National Registry of Emergency Medical Technicians and targeted 1997 for implementation of new examinations that reflect the educational objectives of the new curriculum.

The new curriculum is divided into eight major modules that are further divided into a number of subjects. This review text is divided into sections that correspond to each of the modules. Each section is further divided by the individual subjects contained in each module. The total number of review questions is approximately 350. The distribution of questions among the subjects in each module varies in accordance with the impor-tance of each subject. While certification examinations contain questions on each subject, there are more questions related to life-threatening emergencies than there are for minor medical conditions and administrative matters. The division of the review text allows students to evaluate the areas in which they are weak and need to emphasize during study. This division further allows students to utilize the text during their training course. Use of the review text, during the training course, will allow the students to check on their progress toward achieving certification. Students may request additional help from instructors based on their performance on the review questions.

Each question is in an A-type multiple choice format. This type of question is almost universally used in state and national certifying examinations. There is one correct choice and three distractors for each question. The majority of the questions reflect the new curriculum's emphasis on assessment-based treatment. A brief explanation of the rationale for the correct answer is given for each question. The questions are referenced to information contained in the following textbooks; American Academy of Orothopaedic Surgeons' (A.A.O.S.) *Emergency Care and Transportation of the Sick and Injured,* *Brady's Emergency Care* (7th Edition) and Mosby's *EMT-Basic Textbook.* Each answer has a chapter reference for the corresponding material in the textbooks. This should assist students in studying areas where they need improvement.

We would like to thank Marlene Picone for her administrative assistance, Peter McCurdy for his supervision of the editing of the text and our editor, John Dolan for his enthusiastic support and guidance for this project.

Note

The bibliographic citations following each answer cite the publisher of the book first (Brady, AAOS, or Mosby) and the section or chapter (e.g., Patient Assessment of The Detailed Physical Exam) in that book in which relevant information can be found. For full book information on each citation, please see the Bibliography, on page 129.

EMT-BASIC

PRETEST® SELF-ASSESSMENT AND REVIEW

PREPARATORY

Directions: Each item below contains four suggested responses. Select the **one best** response to each item.

1. The national standards for the EMT-Basic Curriculum are specified by

   (A) the American College of Emergency Physicians
   (B) the United States Department of Transportation
   (C) state governments
   (D) the National Association of EMTs

2. Of the following skills, the one most important for an EMT-Basic to master is

   (A) splinting injured extremities
   (B) coping with a patient's psychological stress
   (C) dressing and bandaging wounds
   (D) providing adequate pulmonary ventilation

3. To qualify for certification as an EMT-Basic, a candidate must generally meet which of the following requirements?

   (A) Successful completion sof a course of instruction that follows the EMT-Basic curriculum
   (B) Age 21 years old or older
   (C) United States citizenship
   (D) High school graduate status

4. Which of the following is a requirement laid down by the Americans with Disabilities Act for the care of disabled persons?

   (A) All ambulances must have wheelchair ramps
   (B) Disabled patients must receive a different level of care than patients without disabilities
   (C) Disabled patients must have equal access to information about their medical conditions
   (D) Disabled patients must be transported to special facilities

5. Which of the following types of prehospital care provider receives the highest level of training?

(A) First Responder
(B) EMT-Basic
(C) EMT-Intermediate
(D) EMT-Paramedic

6. The first responsibility of an EMT-Basic at the scene of an emergency is

(A) the safety of the EMT-Basic, the patient, and others at the scene
(B) appropriate and thorough patient assessment
(C) immediate treatment of life-threatening conditions
(D) safe transportation of the patient to a medical facility

7. An EMT-Basic can best gain a patient's trust and confidence by

(A) speaking in medical terminology
(B) maintaining a professional appearance
(C) asking personal questions
(D) withholding bad news about the patient's condition

8. The systematic review of all aspects of an EMS system is known as

(A) continuing education
(B) medical control
(C) quality improvement
(D) recertification

9. Ensuring that the appropriate care is consistently provided by EMS workers is primarily the responsibility of

(A) ambulance supervisors
(B) the medical director
(C) insurance companies
(D) attorneys

10. The roles and responsibilities of the EMT-Basic include all of the following EXCEPT

(A) the safety of the patient
(B) thorough, accurate patient assessment
(C) safe and efficient patient transport
(D) the restraint of violent patients

11. Which of the following describes the most effective way for EMT personnel to interact with other emergency workers at an emergency site?

(A) EMTs should give orders to public safety workers
(B) EMTs should work independently of other emergency workers
(C) EMTs should work cooperatively with other emergency workers
(D) EMTs should avoid any communication with other emergency workers

12. In relation to an EMS system, quality improvement can best be defined as

(A) a system for identifying areas of an EMS system that need improvement
(B) continuing education of EMS personnel
(C) the purchase of new equipment
(D) improvement in dispatch protocols

13. Ensuring that EMT-Basics provide consistent and appropriate medical care is the responsibility of

(A) the state certifying agency
(B) paramedics
(C) supervisory staff
(D) the medical director

14. All of the following are stages of grief EXCEPT

(A) denial
(B) anger
(C) bargaining
(D) anxiety

15. All of the following could be appropriate in a conversation between an EMT and a patient at the scene of an emergency EXCEPT

(A) honestly discussing the patient's injuries
(B) reassuring a patient that the appropriate help will be provided
(C) assuring the patient that "everything is all right"
(D) explaining what emergency care procedures will be performed

16. Chronic fatigue and job frustration resulting from stress experienced over a period of time is known as

(A) anxiety
(B) irritability
(C) burnout
(D) critical incident stress

17. Which of the following procedures is the most effective for preventing the transmission of disease?

(A) Use of latex gloves
(B) Hand washing
(C) Use of antiseptic solutions
(D) Use of protective clothing

18. Hazardous materials are marked with _____ shaped placards.

(A) circular
(B) square
(C) oval
(D) diamond

19. When an EMT arrives at the scene of a motor vehicle accident where there are fallen electrical power lines, which of the following is an appropriate action for the EMT to take?

(A) Moving the power line using rubber gloves
(B) Turning the power off from the nearest transformer
(C) Establishing a danger zone around the fallen wires
(D) Moving the wires with a wooden pole

20. An EMT-Basic arrives at the scene of a motor vehicle accident, and one of the drivers, who appears to have been drinking, becomes belligerent and threatening. The right course of action for the EMT-Basic is to

(A) attempt to reason with the driver so he doesn't harm anyone or himself
(B) enlist the aid of bystanders to subdue and restrain the driver
(C) leave the scene immediately and not return
(D) retreat to a safe location and call for police assistance

21. When faced with a patient who is unconscious and unable to give consent, an EMT-Basic may provide emergency care under the principle of

(A) expressed consent
(B) informed consent
(C) implied consent
(D) applied consent

22. In the event that a patient refuses emergency medical care, one condition that MUST be satisfied before it is the duty of emergency medical personnel to comply with the patient's refusal is that the patient

(A) have a private physician
(B) have a *Do Not Resuscitate* order
(C) be mentally competent
(D) object to the treatment on religious grounds

23. At the scene of an accident, an injured but obviously competent individual firmly refuses treatment despite the attempts of an EMT to convince him to accept it. The response of the EMT should be to

(A) have the police force the patient to accept treatment
(B) exaggerate the seriousness of the patient's injuries in order to frighten him
(C) simply record that the patient refused treatment on the call report and leave the scene
(D) document the efforts to convince the patient to accept treatment

24. Situations in which an EMT should NOT initiate cardiopulmonary resuscitation on a patient in cardiac arrest include

(A) a patient who has a terminal illness
(B) a patient who has a *Do Not Resuscitate* order
(C) a patient who has a communicable disease
(D) all of the above

25. An EMT-Basic who fails to provide the appropriate standard of care that is expected in a particular situation may be guilty of

(A) assault
(B) battery
(C) abandonment
(D) negligence

26. The most important thing for an EMT-Basic to remember when responding to the scene of a crime is

(A) not to enter the scene
(B) to disturb the scene as little as possible
(C) to wait until patients have left the scene before providing care
(D) to carefully examine all of the objects at the scene

27. The term *anatomic position* is best described by which of the following?

(A) Standing, facing forward, with the arms at the sides and the palms facing forward
(B) Standing, facing forward, with the arms at the sides and the palms facing backward
(C) Lying on the left side
(D) Lying face up

28. The front surface of the body is known as the _____ surface.

(A) anterior
(B) posterior
(C) superior
(D) medial

29. The term *lateral* refers to

(A) areas of the body toward the midline

(B) areas of the body away from the midline

(C) areas toward the rear surface of the body

(D) areas of the body toward the feet

30. The term *proximal* refers to

(A) areas of the body closer to the trunk

(B) areas of the body farther from the trunk

(C) areas toward the front surface of the body

(D) areas of the body toward the head

31. The term *apex* refers to

(A) the top of an anatomic structure

(B) the bottom of an anatomic structure

(C) the largest portion of an anatomic structure

(D) the inner part of an anatomic structure

32. Air entering the respiratory system from the mouth and nose takes which of the following routes?

(A) Epiglottis, pharynx, trachea, larynx, bronchi

(B) Trachea, pharynx, epiglottis, larynx, bronchi

(C) Pharynx, epiglottis, larynx, trachea, bronchi

(D) Larynx, pharynx, trachea, bronchi, epiglottis

33. Which of the following is an important part of the mechanism of normal inhalation?

(A) Contraction of the diaphragm

(B) Relaxation of the diaphragm

(C) Elastic recoil of the lungs

(D) Constriction of the chest cavity

34. In terms of its concentrations of oxygen and carbon dioxide, the blood that enters the lungs from the right side of the heart is best characterized by which of the following statements?

(A) It is high in oxygen and low in carbon dioxide

(B) It is low in both oxygen and carbon dioxide

(C) It is high in both oxygen and carbon dioxide

(D) It is low in oxygen and high in carbon dioxide

35. Blood entering the right atrium will follow which of the following routes?

(A) Right ventricle, pulmonary artery, pulmonary vein, left atrium, left ventricle, aorta

(B) Pulmonary vein, right ventricle, pulmonary artery, left atrium, aorta, left ventricle

(C) Right ventricle, pulmonary vein, pulmonary artery, left atrium, left ventricle, aorta

(D) Aorta, left ventricle, left atrium, pulmonary vein, pulmonary artery, right ventricle

36. The heart muscle is most immediately supplied with oxygenated blood by the

(A) aorta
(B) coronary arteries
(C) pulmonary arteries
(D) superior vena cava

37. The vessel that carries the main supply of blood to the head is the

(A) carotid artery
(B) femoral artery
(C) brachial artery
(D) pulmonary artery

38. Blood is returned toward the heart by blood vessels known as

(A) arteries
(B) capillaries
(C) valves
(D) veins

39. The femoral pulse is an example of which of the following types of pulse?

(A) Peripheral pulse
(B) Central pulse
(C) Distal pulse
(D) Diastolic pulse

40. The autonomic nervous system is responsible for which of the following types of function?

(A) Voluntary motor function
(B) Peripheral sensation
(C) Balance and coordination
(D) Involuntary motor function

41. Which of the following body systems is responsible for secreting the chemical hormones that regulate many bodily functions?

(A) Circulatory system
(B) Nervous system
(C) Respiratory system
(D) Endocrine system

42. The normal pulse rate for an adult at rest is

(A) 50–80 beats per minute
(B) 60–100 beats per minute
(C) 80–110 beats per minute
(D) 100–120 beats per minute

43. The *rhythm* of the pulse refers to the _____ of the pulse.

(A) rate
(B) regularity
(C) strength
(D) location

44. The normal respiratory rate for an adult at rest is

(A) 8–12 breaths per minute
(B) 10–24 breaths per minute
(C) 12–20 breaths per minute
(D) 20–24 breaths per minute

45. Use of the accessory muscles of the shoulders and neck when breathing is a sign of

(A) normal respiration
(B) rapid respiration
(C) quiet respiration
(D) labored respiration

46. Pale skin is a sign of which of the following conditions?

(A) Blood loss
(B) Liver disease
(C) High blood pressure
(D) Lack of oxygen

47. Cool, clammy skin is a sign of which of the following conditions?

(A) Hypothermia
(B) Shock
(C) Fever
(D) Heat exposure

48. When exposed to a bright light, the pupils normally

(A) constrict
(B) dilate
(C) do not change size
(D) become unequal in size

49. Systolic pressure is best defined by which of the following?

(A) The pressure present in the arteries when the heart contracts
(B) The pressure present in the arteries when the heart relaxes
(C) The average of the upper and lower readings obtained when the blood pressure is measured
(D) The difference between the upper and lower readings obtained when the blood pressure is measured

50. A sensation, such as pain or nausea, that a patient describes in relation to a medical condition is an example of a

(A) sign
(B) symptom
(C) vital sign
(D) diagnosis

51. To minimize the chance of aggravating a spinal injury when making an emergency move of a patient, the patient should be moved by being

(A) lifted clear of floor
(B) dragged along the long axis of the body
(C) dragged sideways relative to the long axis of the body
(D) helped to stand and walk

52. The most appropriate device for carrying a patient who has been struck by an auto and is complaining of neck and back pain is the

(A) ambulance cot
(B) stair chair
(C) long spine board
(D) flexible stretcher

PREPARATORY

ANSWERS

1. **The answer is B.** (Brady, Introduction to Emergency Medical Care.) The United States Department of Transportation (DOT) specifies the National Standard Curriculum for EMT-Basic providers. Interested organizations such as the American College of Emergency Physicians and the National Association of EMTs provide advice and input to the Department of Transportation to help develop the curriculum. Individual state governments may require additional training beyond the minimum specified by the Department of Transportation.

2. **The answer is D.** (AAOS, Introduction to Emergency Medical Care.) The ability to provide adequate pulmonary ventilation is an example of care for a life-threatening condition. It is most important for the EMT-Basic to master the skills necessary to care for life-threatening conditions. Splinting of injured extremities, coping with psychological stress, and dressing and bandaging wounds are skills that are used to treat conditions that are not life-threatening.

3. **The answer is A.** (Brady, Introduction to Emergency Medical Care.) To achieve certification as an EMT-Basic, a candidate must successfully complete a course of instruction that follows the National Standard EMT-Basic curriculum. The Department of Transportation does not specify a minimum age of 21. However, many states require a minimum age of 18 for certification as an EMT-Basic. It is not necessary to be a United States citizen or a high school graduate to be certified as an EMT-Basic.

4. **The answer is C.** (AAOS, Introduction to Emergency Medical Care.) The Americans with Disabilities Act requires that disabled patients be kept informed about their medical conditions. Disabled patients must receive an equal level of care as patients without disabilities, and have access to the same medical facilities. No specific equipment is required by the Americans with Disabilities Act.

5. The answer is D. (Brady, Introduction to Emergency Medical Care.) The EMT-Paramedic completes an extensive course in advanced life support and attains the highest level of training of any prehospital care provider. First Responders are the first trained persons to respond to the scene of an emergency. Most first responders are police officers and firefighters, who are trained to assess the situation and provide simple lifesaving treatments, such as CPR and bleeding control. The EMT-Basic receives more extensive training in patient assessment and basic life support. The EMT-Intermediate receives training in specific areas of advanced life support, such as IV therapy and the interpretation of cardiac rhythms.

6. The answer is A. (AAOS, Introduction to Emergency Medical Care.) The first responsibility of an EMT-Basic is to maintain safety at the scene. Patient assessment, treatment, and transportation are all important responsibilities, but the EMT-Basic must first establish a safe environment at the scene so that there are no further injuries.

7. The answer is B. (AAOS, Introduction to Emergency Medical Care.) A professional appearance will help the patient to be confident of the EMT-Basic's ability. EMT-Basics should have a basic knowledge of medical terminology but should always address the patient with language and terms that will be understood. It is not appropriate to ask personal questions unless they relate to the patient's medical condition. The EMT-Basic must always keep patients informed of their condition.

8. The answer is C. (Brady, Introduction to Emergency Medical Care.) *Quality improvement* is the systematic review of all aspects of an EMS system for the purpose of identifying areas that need improvement. *Medical control* is the direction provided by the physician medical director. *Continuing education* allows EMT-Basics to keep their knowledge and skills up to date. Many states require that EMT-Basics undergo periodic *recertification* to ensure that their knowledge and skills are up to date.

9. The answer is B. (AAOS, Introduction to Emergency Medical Care.) The physician medical director is the person primarily responsible for the quality of the medical care delivered by EMS workers. Trained supervisory personnel may assist the medical director in this task. Insurance companies and attorneys are not responsible for the quality of medical care provided.

10. The answer is D. (Brady, Introduction to Emergency Medical Care.) EMTs are primarily responsible for maintaining a safe working environment at the scene of an emergency, assessing patients for medical problems, rendering patient care at the scene, and transporting patients to a medical facility in an appropriate manner. The restraint of violent or uncooperative patients is the responsibility of law enforcement officers, who are better trained and equipped for this type of activity.

11. The answer is C. (AAOS, Introduction to Emergency Medical Care.) EMTs are part of a system that is designed to deliver emergency care to those in need. Other emergency workers, such as firefighters, are often trained to deliver emergency care. EMTs must work cooperatively with these other emergency workers to achieve the best outcome for the patient. Good lines of communication must be established at the scene of an emergency to provide patients with the best emergency care.

12. The answer is A. (Brady, Introduction to Emergency Medical Care.) *Quality improvement* is a system for collecting data in an organized manner to identify which areas of an EMS system need improvement. Quality improvement may identify the need for such specific actions as continuing education, replacement of old equipment, or the institution of more accurate dispatch procedures.

13. The answer is D. (Brady, Introduction to Emergency Medical Care.) The medical director is responsible for the overall quality of medical care that EMT-Basics deliver to patients at the scene of an emergency by establishing treatment protocols and reviewing the care rendered by EMT-Basics. State certifying agencies ensure that those persons certified as EMT-Basics have the appropriate training and the necessary skills. Paramedics may assist with EMT training and direct the actions of EMTs at the scene of an emergency in accordance with the medical director's instructions. Supervisors are primarily concerned with administrative matters.

14. The answer is D. (AAOS, The well being of the EMT-B.) The grieving process for most individuals follows a predictable pattern. Survivors first tend to *deny* their loss. Once the loss is recognized, a period of *anger* often follows. *Bargaining* is an attempt by survivors to minimize the impact of the loss. The final stage of grief is an *acceptance* of the loss and a desire to move on. Anxiety is a response to any type of stress, and not a stage of grief.

15. The answer is C. (AAOS, The well being of the EMT-B.) When speaking with an injured patient, the EMT must always be honest. Statements such as "everything is all right" should be avoided—a patient who has just wrecked a new car and is in severe pain knows that everything is not all right. Patients should be reassured that the appropriate medical care will be provided. Explaining an emergency care procedure to a patient before performing it will help to gain the patient's confidence and cooperation.

16. The answer is C. (AAOS, The well being of the EMT-B.) *Burnout* is a condition caused by long-term stress. It is characterized by increasing frustration with work and chronic fatigue. Burnout is common among health-care and emergency workers. *Anxiety*, on the other hand, is an immediate reaction to an acute stress. *Irritability* is often apparent in those who are under great stress. *Critical incident stress* is a response to a particular incident that the EMT finds overwhelming. Typical situations that generate critical incident stress are multiple casualty incidents, badly injured patients, and incidents involving children.

17. The answer is B. (Mosby, The well being of the EMT-B.) Hand washing is the most effective procedure for preventing the transmission of disease. EMTs should wash their hands thoroughly before and after every patient contact. This is important even when barriers such as latex gloves and protective clothing have been used. The hands are the most common means of spreading infectious diseases. Gloves may leak and do not always provide complete protection. Antiseptic solutions may be helpful but are not as effective as vigorous hand washing with soap and water.

18. The answer is D. (Mosby, The well being of the EMT-B.) Hazardous materials are marked with colored, diamond-shaped placards. The placards have an international symbol and lettering that identifies the general type of hazard. Some materials are also identified by a number that can be checked in the Department of Transportation publication *Hazardous Materials: The Emergency Response Book.*

19. The answer is C. (AAOS, The well being of the EMT-B.) Dealing with downed power lines is beyond the training of the EMT-Basic. Special training and equipment are necessary to deal with electrical power lines. Use of insulated gloves and special wooden poles should be left to specially trained individuals. Only power company employees should attempt to shut power off. EMT-Basics should call for assistance from the power company and make no attempt to move downed power lines. A danger zone should be established around the fallen lines, and access to this area limited strictly to essential personnel. Utility poles may be used as landmarks for establishing the perimeter of the danger zone.

20. The answer is D. (Brady, The well being of the EMT-B.) When faced with a potentially violent situation, the EMT-Basic should retreat to a safe location and radio for police assistance. It is often not possible to reason with an intoxicated individual. The EMT-Basic is not properly trained or equipped to subdue or restrain a violent individual. The police are properly trained and authorized to deal with violent situations. It is not appropriate for the EMT-Basic to just leave the scene, as that could amount to abandoning patients who need medical assistance.

21. The answer is C. (AAOS, Medical-Legal Issues.) It is assumed that the patient would consent to treatment if able to do so. This is known as *implied consent. Expressed consent* occurs when a competent patient actually gives consent to receive treatment. For a patient to give *informed consent*, the EMT-Basic must explain all of the benefits and potential risks of the treatment. An EMT-Basic should attempt to obtain informed consent whenever possible.

22. The answer is C. (AAOS, Medical-Legal Issues.) A patient must be mentally competent and not have any condition that would impair judgment in order to legally refuse emergency care. The patient must be able to understand the potential consequences of refusing care. A patient need not have a private physician to refuse emergency care, but patients who refuse care should be encouraged to consult a physician as soon as possible. A *Do Not Resuscitate* order applies only to cardiopulmonary resuscitation. Patients may refuse emergency treatment for a variety of reasons, religious and otherwise.

23. The answer is D. (Brady, Medical-Legal Issues.) It is important for the EMT to document the attempts to convince the patient to accept treatment, as well as the names of any witnesses to these efforts. This record is important in case the patient's condition should deteriorate as a result of his or her decision. Inadequate documentation may not protect the EMT from liability. In most cases, no one is entitled to force a competent person to accept medical treatment. An EMT should always be truthful with a patient when discussing the patient's medical condition.

24. The answer is B. (Brady, Medical-Legal Issues.) Unless there is positive evidence of death, such as decomposition, rigor mortis, lividity, or obvious mortal injury, an EMT should initiate cardiopulmonary resuscitation on all patients in cardiac arrest unless a *Do Not Resuscitate* order is in effect. The presence of a terminal illness is not a contraindication to cardiopulmonary resuscitation. An EMT must take precautions against the spread of communicable diseases whenever performing cardiopulmonary resuscitation.

25. The answer is D. (AAOS, Medical-Legal Issues.) An EMT-Basic who has a duty to act and fails to act in accordance with the standard of care may be found negligent. To prove negligence, it is further necessary to show that the patient suffered some injury as a direct result of the failure of the EMT-Basic to provide the appropriate standard of care. *Assault* and *battery* refer to the unauthorized threatening and touching of an individual. *Abandonment* occurs when an EMT-Basic suddenly terminates the treatment of a patient who still requires treatment.

26. The answer is B. (AAOS, Medical-Legal Issues.) If there are any patients at a crime scene, the EMT-Basic must enter the scene and provide the appropriate emergency care, both at the scene and during transportation of the patients. The EMT-Basic should attempt to disturb the scene as little as possible so as not to destroy or obscure any evidence that may be present. The EMT-Basic should not handle or move any objects at the scene unless doing so is necessary for the treatment of the patient.

27. The answer is A. (Brady, The Human Body.) The anatomic position is a standard posture of reference for describing the relationship between areas of the body. This standard is necessary so that all areas of the body will be described in a like manner. In the anatomic position, the body is standing face forward, with the arms at the sides and palms facing forward. Regardless of a patient's actual position, all areas on the body are described as though the patient were in the anatomic position.

28. The answer is A. (Mosby, The Human Body.) The term *anterior* refers to the front surface of the body. *Posterior* refers to the rear surface of the body, also called the *dorsal surface*. *Superior* describes anatomic structures that are above other structures of the body. *Medial* describes structures that are toward the midline of the body. All location descriptions are based on a body in the anatomic position.

29. The answer is B. (Mosby, The Human Body.) The term *lateral* is a relative anatomic term used to describe areas of the body that are farther from the midline when the body is in the anatomic position. For example, the ears can be said to be lateral to the eyes, because they are farther from the midline of the body than the eyes.

30. The answer is A. (Mosby, The Human Body.) The term *proximal* is a relative anatomic term used to describe areas of the body that are closer to the trunk when the body is in the anatomic position. This term is most commonly used by EMTs to describe areas on limbs. For example, the knee is proximal to the ankle because it is closer to the trunk than is the ankle.

31. The answer is A. (Brady, The Human Body.) The term *apex* refers to the top (most superior aspect) of an anatomic structure. (The term *superior* means farther toward the top.) For example, the top portion of the lung is called the apex of the lung. All these terms are used to describe the body in the anatomic position.

32. The answer is C. (Brady, The Human Body.) Air entering through the mouth or nose first reaches the pharynx, which is the area directly posterior to the mouth and nose. The air then passes the epiglottis, which is the structure that prevents food and foreign objects from entering the larynx (also known as the voice box). Air then moves into the trachea, which splits into the right and left mainstem bronchi.

33. The answer is A. (Brady, The Human Body.) The diaphragm is a muscle located at the bottom of the chest cavity. During normal inhalation, the diaphragm contracts, moving downward and causing the chest cavity to expand. This expansion draws external air into the lungs. During exhalation, the diaphragm relaxes, and the elastic recoil of the lungs expels the air, causing the chest cavity to become smaller.

34. The answer is D. (AAOS, The Human Body.) Blood that has given up oxygen to the cells of the body and taken up carbon dioxide returns to the right side of the heart. From the right side of the heart, this blood—low in oxygen and high in carbon dioxide—is pumped to the lungs, where it takes up oxygen from the inspired air and releases carbon dioxide.

35. The answer is A. (AAOS, The Human Body.) After entering the right atrium, blood passes through the tricuspid valve into the right ventricle. From the right ventricle, it is pumped out through the pulmonary artery into the lungs. Blood returns through the pulmonary veins into the left atrium. It then passes through the mitral valve into the left ventricle. From the left ventricle, it is pumped out through the aorta to the rest of the body.

36. The answer is B. (Brady, The Human Body.) The coronary arteries supply oxygenated blood to the heart muscle. If there is a blockage in one of the coronary arteries, there may be damage to the heart muscle. This may result in a heart attack. The aorta is the main artery that supplies blood to the rest of the body. (The coronary arteries originate from the base of the aorta.) The pulmonary arteries take deoxygenated blood from the right ventricle to the lungs. The superior vena cava returns blood from the upper part of the body to the right atrium.

37. **The answer is A.** (Brady, The Human Body.) The carotid artery is the large artery in the neck that carries most of the blood supply for the head. The carotid artery is palpated for the presence of a pulse during CPR. The femoral artery supplies blood to the leg. The brachial artery supplies blood to the forearm. The pulmonary arteries take deoxygenated blood from the right ventricle to the lungs.

38. **The answer is D.** (Brady, The Human Body.) Veins are vessels that return blood from the body tissues toward the heart. Veins begin at the capillaries as tiny vessels known as venules. Capillaries are tiny blood vessels whose walls are so thin that oxygen, carbon dioxide, nutrients, and waste products can be exchanged between the blood and the cells. The arteries carry blood away from the heart. Valves are structures within the heart and circulatory system that ensure that blood flows in the correct direction.

39. **The answer is B.** (Brady, The Human Body.) The femoral artery is a large vessel in the groin. Since the femoral pulse can be felt in the central area of the body, it is called a *central pulse. Peripheral* and *distal pulses* are those that can be felt on the extremities. Because central pulses are felt in large vessels that are near the heart, they can often be felt when the peripheral or distal pulses are too weak to palpate.

40. **The answer is D.** (Brady, The Human Body.) The autonomic nervous system is a branch of the peripheral nervous system that controls involuntary motor functions such as heart rate, blood pressure, and control of the digestive system.

41. **The answer is D.** (AAOS, The Human Body.) The endocrine glands secrete specialized chemicals known as hormones into the bloodstream. Insulin and epinephrine are examples of hormones, regulating such body functions as the metabolism of sugar and the heart rate and blood pressure.

42. **The answer is B.** (AAOS, Vital Signs and Patient History.) The normal resting pulse rate for adults is 60 to 100 beats per minute. Pulse rates below 60 beats per minute are usually considered slow, although they may be normal for athletic individuals. The term for an abnormally slow pulse rate is *bradycardia*. Pulse rates above 100 beats per minute are considered fast. An abnormally fast pulse rate is known as *tachycardia*.

43. **The answer is B.** (AAOS, Vital Signs and Patient History.) The rhythm of the pulse refers to the regularity of the pulse. The EMT-Basic should assess the rhythm of every patient's pulse. A pulse should normally be regular, having a constant interval between each beat. An irregular pulse, in which the interval between beats is variable, may be an indication of cardiac disease.

44. **The answer is C.** (AAOS, Vital Signs and Patient History.) While respiratory rate varies greatly with differences in size, physical condition, and level of anxiety, most adults breathe at approximately 12 to 20 breaths per minute when at rest. The EMT-Basic should administer oxygen and consider artificial ventilation for any patient with a respiratory rate of less than 8 or greater than 24 breaths per minute.

45. The answer is D. (AAOS, Vital Signs and Patient History.) Patients who are in respiratory distress with labored respiration will attempt to use the accessory muscles of the neck and shoulders to expand the chest and bring more air into the lungs. It is useful to look for use of these muscles when assessing a patient for the presence of respiratory distress.

46. The answer is A. (Brady, Baseline Vital Signs.) Patients with blood loss often appear pale, as do those with constricted blood vessels due to shock, heart attack, or anxiety. Liver disease often causes a yellowish discoloration of the skin known as *jaundice*. Patients with high blood pressure generally appear flushed. A lack of oxygen causes a bluish discoloration of the skin known as *cyanosis*.

47. The answer is B. (Brady, Baseline Vital Signs.) Patients in shock usually are cool and clammy to the touch because of the constriction of the blood vessels in the skin. Hypothermia causes the skin to feel cool and dry. Fever causes the skin to feel warm. Patients often can be assessed for fever by feeling the skin. Heat exposure also makes the skin feel warm.

48. The answer is A. (Mosby, Baseline Vital Signs.) The function of the pupils is to regulate the amount of light entering the eye by dilating (to admit more light) and constricting (to admit less light). When exposed to bright light, a normal pupil constricts. Pupils that are unreactive to light may be a sign of hypoxia, drug use, or brain injury. Unequal pupils (pupils of unequal size) may be a sign of brain injury or injury to the eye.

49. The answer is A. (Brady, Baseline Vital Signs.) The pressure that is present in the arteries when the heart contracts is the *systolic pressure*, whereas the pressure that is present when the heart is relaxed is the *diastolic pressure*. Both these pressures are obtained during a blood pressure measurement. While air is being released gradually from the pressure cuff, the pressure shown by the pressure gauge at the moment sounds are first heard through the stethoscope is the systolic pressure, and the pressure shown by the gauge at the moment sounds disappear is the diastolic pressure.

50. The answer is B. (AAOS, Vital Signs and Patient History.) Both symptoms and signs are pieces of evidence about a medical condition. A *symptom* is a piece of evidence that cannot be directly observed by another person but can be perceived and reported by the patient. An example is chest pain. A *sign* is a piece of evidence that can be observed or measured directly by another person. Unequal pupil diameter is an example.

51. The answer is B. (AAOS, Lifting and Moving Patients.) When making an emergency move of a patient, the safest maneuver is to drag the patient along the long axis of the body. This method will allow the spine to assume its normal position. Attempting to lift the patient or have the patient stand will cause a considerable amount of flexion and twisting of the spine. Dragging the patient sideways will pull the spine out of its normal alignment.

52. The answer is C. (Brady, Lifting and Moving Patients.) A spinal injury must be suspected in a patient who complains of neck or back pain after an injury. The long spine board allows the patient's spine to be immobilized more effectively than any of the other devices.

AIRWAY

Directions: Each item below contains four suggested responses. Select the **one best** response to each item.

53. The most appropriate treatment for an unresponsive patient with occasional gasping respirations is

    (A) artificial ventilation with supplemental oxygen
    (B) ventilation with a non-rebreather with oxygen at 10 liters per minute
    (C) ventilation with a nasal cannula with oxygen at 6 liters per minute
    (D) immediate transport

54. The simplest method of establishing and maintaining an airway in an unresponsive patient who has not suffered any trauma is

    (A) head tilt and chin lift
    (B) the modified jaw thrust
    (C) an oropharyngeal airway
    (D) nasopharyngeal airway

55. Adult patients should be suctioned for no more than ____ seconds.

    (A) 5
    (B) 15
    (C) 20
    (D) 30

56. Which of the following distances on a patient can be used to determine the correct depth for insertion of a soft suction catheter?

    (A) From the corner of the mouth to the ear
    (B) From the corner of the mouth to the Adam's apple
    (C) From the tip of the nose to the ear
    (D) From the tip of the nose to the Adam's apple

57. A high-pitched wheezing sound heard on expiration when listening to the chest is an indication of

(A) fluid in the lungs
(B) constricted bronchi
(C) pneumonia
(D) partial upper airway obstruction

58. You listen to a patient's chest with your stethoscope and find that there are no breath sounds in one area of the chest. This finding is an indication of

(A) fluid in the lungs
(B) complete upper airway obstruction
(C) lack of air movement
(D) moderate bronchoconstriction

59. How should an uninjured patient who is breathing spontaneously be positioned to keep the airway clear of secretion or vomitus?

(A) Lying supine
(B) Lying prone
(C) Lying on one side
(D) With the head elevated

60. A single EMT-Basic can most effectively provide artificial ventilation by which of the following methods?

(A) Mouth-to-mouth ventilation
(B) Mouth-to mask ventilation
(C) Bag-valve-mask ventilation
(D) Use of an oxygen-powered breathing device

61. Without the use of supplemental oxygen, mouth-to-mouth or mouth-to-mask ventilation will deliver which of the following oxygen concentrations?

(A) 12%
(B) 16%
(C) 21%
(D) 24%

62. The primary disadvantage of the bag-valve-mask method for artificial ventilation is

(A) the difficulty of maintaining a tight seal with the mask
(B) the inability to provide a high concentration of oxygen
(C) the weight and complexity of the unit
(D) the fact that the method can only be used on patients who are not breathing spontaneously

63. A bag-valve-mask device should have all of the following features EXCEPT

(A) A one-way valve
(B) A transparent face mask
(C) An oxygen reservoir
(D) A pop-off valve

64. Which of the following is a specific sign of complete obstruction of the airway by a foreign body?

(A) A forceful cough
(B) Cyanosis
(C) A sudden inability to speak or cough occurring while the patient is eating
(D) Rapid, gasping respirations

65. Use of an oropharyngeal airway is appropriate for some conditions in all of the following patient groups EXCEPT

(A) responsive patients
(B) patients less than 8 years old
(C) patients requiring artificial ventilation
(D) patients less than 5 feet tall

66. Which of the following distances on a patient can be used to determine the correct size of oropharyngeal airway for use in that patient?

(A) From the tip of the nose to the ear
(B) From the corner of the mouth to the ear lobe
(C) From the corner of the mouth to the Adam's apple
(D) From tip of the nose to the corner of the mouth

67. Which of the following is a major advantage of the nasopharyngeal airway?

(A) It can be used for responsive patients
(B) It protects the airway from vomiting
(C) It will prevent nosebleeds
(D) It does not require lubrication

68. In terms of supplemental oxygen, patients with inadequate breathing should always receive

(A) no supplemental oxygen
(B) a low concentration of supplemental oxygen
(C) a high concentration of supplemental oxygen
(D) just enough supplemental oxygen to cause the patient's color to improve

69. Which of the following devices will deliver the highest concentration of oxygen to a spontaneously breathing patient?

(A) Simple face mask
(B) Nasal cannula
(C) Non-rebreather mask
(D) Venturi mask

AIRWAY

ANSWERS

53. The answer is A. (AAOS, Mechanics of Breathing) Occasional gasping respirations are seen in patients who are near death. They are known as *agonal respirations* and precede the complete cessation of breathing. Agonal respirations are always inadequate, and artificial ventilation is necessary. Oxygen delivery devices, such as the non-rebreather or nasal cannula, are ineffective because there is insufficient air exchange. Ventilation must be established prior to transport.

54. The answer is A. (AAOS, Airway and Ventilation) Tilting the head back while lifting the chin will establish an airway quickly and easily and is appropriate in an unresponsive patient with no history of trauma. This method is easy to learn and requires no equipment. The modified jaw thrust requires more training; it should be used for patients with suspected cervical spine trauma. Use of the oropharyngeal and nasopharyngeal airways requires more training and the use of equipment.

55. The answer is B. (AAOS, Airway and Ventilation) It is necessary to stop ventilations in order to suction a patient's airway. Suctioning, therefore, should be limited to 15 seconds. If the airway cannot be cleared with 15 seconds of suctioning, the patient should be rolled to one side and the airway cleared manually. Children should be suctioned for even shorter times, because they have a smaller respiratory reserve.

56. The answer is C. (Brady, Airway Management) To suction most effectively, the tip of the catheter should be placed at the base of the tongue. The depth of insertion should be measured from the tip of the nose to the ear. Insertion to this length will position the tip of the catheter appropriately at the base of the tongue.

57. The answer is B. (Brady, Airway Management) High-pitched sounds heard over the chest on expiration are known as wheezes. Wheezes are an indication of constricted bronchi. Constriction of the bronchi is caused by lung diseases such as asthma and bronchitis. Fluid in the lungs will produce a lower-pitched crackling sound. Pneumonia will produce crackling sounds and areas of absent breath sounds. A high-pitched sound heard over the trachea on inspiration is an indication of upper airway obstruction.

58. **The answer is C.** (Brady, The Focused History and Physical Exam—The Trauma Patient) The movement of air through the lungs produces sounds that can be heard over the chest with a stethoscope. The absence of sound over an area of the chest indicates that no air is moving through the underlying region of lung. The lung may have collapsed beneath that area, or the patient may have a pneumonia that is preventing air from entering the area. Fluid in the lungs will produce crackling sounds. Bronchoconstriction is identified by high-pitched wheezes that are heard on expiration. In patients with complete airway obstruction, breath sounds are absent over the entire chest.

59. **The answer is C.** (AAOS, Airway and Ventilation) Patients who are breathing spontaneously and have no traumatic injury can be placed lying on one side to allow secretions or vomitus to drain away from the airway. Care must be taken if a head or spinal injury is suspected. In such cases, the patient can be carefully rolled as a unit onto one side, with the head and spine kept in line.

60. **The answer is B.** (Brady, Airway Management) The mouth-to-mask technique of artificial ventilation is the most effective method for an EMT-Basic who is working alone. The mask and one-way valve are simple and light and can easily be brought to the scene. The EMT-Basic can use both hands to achieve a tight seal against the patient's face. Many mouth-to-mask units allow for the use of enriched oxygen concentrations by the addition of supplemental oxygen to the unit. Mouth-to-mouth ventilation should always be performed with an appropriate barrier device. It is sometime difficult to obtain an adequate seal with these barrier devices. A single EMT-Basic will have difficulty achieving the tight seal necessary to effectively use the bag-valve-mask or oxygen-powered breathing device with one hand.

61. **The answer is B.** (AAOS, Airway and Ventilation) Atmospheric air contains 21% oxygen. The exhaled air that is delivered to a patient who is receiving mouth-to-mouth or mouth-to-mask ventilation contains 16% oxygen. Supplemental oxygen may be added to many mouth-to-mask units. Adding supplemental oxygen to a mouth-to-mask unit can increase the oxygen concentration up to approximately 55%.

62. **The answer is A.** (Brady, Airway Management) It is difficult to maintain a tight seal with the mask of the bag-valve-mask device. It is especially difficult for a single EMT to maintain an adequate seal with one hand while squeezing the bag with the other. Whenever possible, two persons should operate the bag-valve-mask device, one maintaining the seal with two hands while the other squeezes the bag. The bag-valve-mask is a simple, lightweight device that can use supplemental oxygen. It may be used to assist the ventilation of a spontaneously breathing patient.

63. The answer is D. (Mosby, The Airway) A bag valve mask should have a one-way valve to prevent the patient from inhaling any exhaled air; a transparent face mask to allow the EMT to monitor the patient for the presence of vomiting, and an oxygen reservoir to allow for the delivery of a high concentration of oxygen when the device is used with supplemental oxygen.

64. The answer is C. (AAOS, Airway and Ventilation) Most foreign-body airway obstructions involve food and occur immediately after a bite is eaten. A patient with a complete foreign-body airway obstruction will not be able to move enough air to speak or cough. Cyanosis is seen in many conditions that cause the patient to be deficient in oxygen and thus is not a specific sign. Patients with a complete foreign-body airway obstruction will not be able to breathe at all.

65. The answer is A. (Mosby, The Airway) Responsive patients cannot tolerate an oropharyngeal airway because it will stimulate a gag reflex. Inserting an oropharyngeal airway into a responsive patient may cause retching or vomiting. Oropharyngeal airways are available in various sizes for patients of all sizes and ages. They are useful for maintaining an open airway in patients receiving artificial ventilation.

66. The answer is B. (AAOS, Airway Adjuncts and Oxygen Equipment) Oropharyngeal airways are available in various sizes to fit all patients from infants to large adults. The appropriate size of airway for a particular patient can be selected by comparing the airway to the distance from the corner of the patient's mouth to the patient's ear lobe. If the airway is the right size, its flange should rest at the lips when it is inserted.

67. The answer is A. (AAOS, Airway Adjuncts and Oxygen Equipment) Nasopharyngeal airways are usually tolerated by responsive patients and will not cause the retching or vomiting associated with oropharyngeal airways. Although nasopharyngeal airways will not cause vomiting, they will not protect the airway if the patient vomits for other reasons. Nasopharyngeal airways should always be lubricated with a water-soluble lubricant. Nosebleeds are a complication of the nasopharyngeal airway.

68. The answer is C. (Brady, Airway Management) Patients with inadequate breathing should receive the highest possible concentration of oxygen. These patients are severely hypoxic and require artificial ventilation. Whenever possible, high-concentration oxygen should be added to the device used to deliver artificial ventilation.

69. The answer is C. (AAOS, Airway Adjuncts and Oxygen Equipment) The non-rebreather mask with a good seal around the mask and nose can provide oxygen concentrations of up to 95% to a spontaneously breathing patient. The nasal cannula can provide low to moderate concentrations (24% to 50%) depending on the oxygen flow. The simple face mask and the venturi mask provide moderate concentrations of oxygen, but they are not commonly used in the prehospital setting.

PATIENT ASSESSMENT

Directions: Each item below contains four suggested responses. Select the **one best** response to each item.

70. The FIRST responsibility of an EMT-Basic when arriving at an emergency scene is to

(A) assess any patients for life-threatening injuries
(B) begin treating any life-threatening problems
(C) call for additional units if necessary
(D) identify any hazards that are present at the scene

71. Which of the following is the best question to ask to ascertain a patient's chief complaints?

(A) Are you all right?
(B) Do you have any medical problems?
(C) Do you have chest pain?
(D) Why did you call for help today?

72. The main purpose of the primary survey is to

(A) identify any medical problems
(B) find the chief complaint
(C) identify and correct any life-threatening conditions
(D) determine the patient's past medical history

73. What is the first step in assessing the adequacy of a patient's airway?

(A) Determining the level of consciousness
(B) Assessing breath sounds
(C) Determining the past medical history
(D) Finding if the patient can speak

74. The most effective way to initially assess an unresponsive patient for the presence of breathing is to

(A) listen for the presence of breath sounds
(B) look, listen, and feel for air exchange
(C) assess the patient for cyanosis
(D) hold a mirror near the patient's mouth and nose and observe for fogging

75. The most common location for assessing the pulse of a responsive patient is

(A) the carotid pulse in the neck
(B) the femoral pulse in the groin
(C) the brachial pulse in the arm
(D) the radial pulse in the wrist

76. The presence of a radial pulse usually indicates that the patient's systolic blood pressure is at least

(A) 60 mm Hg
(B) 80 mm Hg
(C) 100 mm Hg
(D) 120 mm Hg

77. The carotid pulse can best be palpated in which of the following locations?

(A) Just beneath the Adam's apple
(B) On either side of the spine
(C) Between the Adam's apple and muscles on the side of the neck
(D) Just beneath the angle of the jaw

78. You cannot feel a pulse, but you suspect that the patient has a heartbeat. Which of the following should you do?

(A) Start CPR
(B) Check for an apical pulse by listening over the left side of the patient's chest
(C) Attach the automated external defibrillator to check the patient's heart rhythm
(D) Check capillary refill

79. If the patient's condition permits, a head-to-toe assessment of a trauma patient should be performed at which of the following points in the course of emergency care?

(A) As soon as the EMT arrives
(B) After life-threatening conditions have been identified and stabilized
(C) Only while en route to the hospital
(D) Only after arrival at the hospital

80. If the primary survey reveals that a trauma patient is having difficulty breathing, the EMT-Basic should

(A) first complete the head-to-toe assessment and then administer high-concentration oxygen
(B) first administer high-concentration oxygen and then complete the head-to-toe assessment
(C) transport the patient with no further assessment or treatment
(D) first administer high-concentration oxygen, then begin transport and complete the head-to-toe assessment while en route to the hospital

81. When assessing and stabilizing the airway of an unresponsive trauma patient, the EMT-Basic should

(A) immediately open the airway by the head-tilt/jaw-lift method
(B) keep the cervical spine in line and use the modified jaw thrust
(C) turn the patient's head to the side to allow blood and secretions to drain
(D) use the Heimlich manuever to clear blood or secretions

82. A light crackling sensation felt over the surface of the chest is an indication of

(A) normal breathing
(B) inadequate breathing
(C) a fractured rib
(D) rupture of the lung or air passages

83. The presence of decreased breath sounds in a trauma patient is an indication of

(A) normal breathing
(B) complete airway obstruction
(C) injury to the lung
(D) shock

84. In a patient with a medical problem, the EMT-Basic should assess the level of consciousness every _____ minutes.

(A) 2
(B) 10
(C) 30
(D) 60

85. Which of the following is the largest (most inclusive) group of patients on whom a rapid trauma assessment should be done?

(A) All patients
(B) Any patient who has a mechanism of trauma that indicates severe injury
(C) All patients over 65 years old
(D) Any patient complaining of neck pain

86. If a life-threatening condition is identified during patient assessment, the EMT-Basic should proceed by

(A) immediately dealing with the life-threatening condition
(B) completing the assessment and then treating the condition
(C) noting the condition on the call report
(D) immediately beginning transport and treating the condition en route to the hospital

87. How long should the rapid trauma assessment take?

(A) Less than 1 minute
(B) 1 to 2 minutes
(C) 5 minutes
(D) 10 minutes

88. Upon examining a patient's chest, you note that one area moves in the opposite direction from the rest. This phenomenon is known as

(A) unequal respiration
(B) paradoxical respiration
(C) disturbed respiration
(D) labored respiration

89. In most cases, the detailed physical examination should be performed at which of the following points in the course of emergency care?

(A) At the scene, prior to transport
(B) While en route to the hospital
(C) Prior to any treatment
(D) Only at the hospital

PATIENT ASSESSMENT

70. The answer is D. (Mosby, Scene Size Up) The first duty of an EMT-Basic on arriving at a scene is to survey it for hazards such as traffic, fire, hazardous materials, or violent individuals. This step precedes assessment or treatment of patients. Rescue workers that are unaware of hazards present at an emergency scene are likely to become additional victims. After identifying any hazards, the EMT-Basic should call for any additional assistance that may be necessary.

71. The answer is D. (AAOS, Scene Size Up and Initial Assessment) The *chief complaint* is the symptom that is most troubling to the patient. Ascertaining the chief complaint at the start of the assessment helps the EMT-Basic to focus on the patient's present problem. The best way to do this is to ask the patient why he or she called for help. Specific questions that may be answered with a yes or no, such as "Are you all right" or "Do you have chest pain," will not help to reveal the chief complaint. Immediately asking questions about past medical problems may obscure the present problem.

72. The answer is C. (AAOS, Scene Size Up and Initial Assessment) The EMT-Basic must immediately assess every patient for the presence of any life threatening problems. The primary concern is to identify and, if possible, correct any threat to the patient's airway, breathing, circulation, or nervous system. After life-threatening conditions have been corrected, the EMT-Basic can go on to determine the patient's chief complaint and past medical history and can perform a more complete assessment.

73. The answer is A. (AAOS, Scene Size Up and Initial Assessment) The most common cause of airway obstruction is the tongue falling back into the oropharynx. The muscles that normally hold the tongue in position are relaxed in patients who are unconscious, allowing the tongue to move posteriorly and block the airway. The EMT-Basic should first determine the patient's level of consciousness by the assessing the patient's responsiveness to verbal and tactile stim-

27

ulation. Patients who are not responsive are at risk for airway obstruction. Responsive patients should be assessed for the ability to speak. Breath sounds may be affected by many factors other than airway obstruction.

74. **The answer is B.** (AAOS, Scene Size Up and Initial Assessment) The quickest and most effective way to determine if an unresponsive patient is breathing is to look for chest movement while listening and feeling for air movement at the patient's mouth and nose. Listening for breath sounds requires more time and equipment. Looking for the absence of cyanosis or the presence of fogging on a mirror held near the patient's mouth and nose are not reliable methods of assessing a patient for the presence of breathing.

75. **The answer is D.** (AAOS, Scene Size Up and Initial Assessment) The most accessible location for assessing the pulse of a responsive patient is the wrist. It is not necessary to remove any clothing or position the patient in any way to assess the radial pulse. Patients often find the touching supplied while taking a radial pulse reassuring. It is usually necessary to remove clothing to assess brachial and femoral pulses. Carotid pulses should be assessed in all patients who are unresponsive.

76. **The answer is B.** (AAOS, Scene Size Up and Initial Assessment) In most cases, the presence of a radial pulse indicates a systolic blood pressure of at least 80 mm Hg. If a radial pulse cannot be palpated in either of the patient's wrists, an attempt should be made to palpate a carotid pulse to determine the patient's heart rate and rhythm. The carotid pulse is easier to palpate in a patient with low blood pressure. The presence of a carotid pulse indicates a systolic blood pressure of at least 60 mm Hg.

77. **The answer is C.** (AAOS, Scene Size Up and Initial Assessment) The carotid pulse is best located by placing the fingers gently on the patient's Adam's apple and moving them to either side until the pulse is felt in the area between the Adam's apple and neck muscle.

78. **The answer is B.** (AAOS, Scene Size Up and Initial Assessment) In some cases, a pulse cannot be palpated despite the presence of a heartbeat. The heartbeat may be suggested by the presence of breathing or other signs of life. Initiating CPR on a patient with a heartbeat may cause cardiac arrest. In these cases, you should listen over the left side of the patient's chest with a stethoscope. If there is any cardiac activity, you will hear heart sounds. Capillary refill is not always a reliable sign of the presence or absence of a pulse. The automated external defibrillator (AED) can detect electrical activity but not the presence or absence of an effective heartbeat.

79. **The answer is B.** (AAOS, Patient Assessment) The EMT-Basic must complete the primary survey before beginning a complete head-to-toe assessment. Any life-threatening problems that are identified during the primary survey must be stabilized before any further examination is attempted. If life-threatening conditions cannot be stabilized, the patient should be transported immediately. A head-to-toe survey can be conducted en route to the hospital if necessary.

80. **The answer is D.** (AAOS, Patient Assessment) Difficulty with breathing in a trauma patient may be a sign of a serious underlying condition that will require immediate hospital treatment. The EMT-Basic should immediately administer high-concentration oxygen to help stabilize the patient's breathing. Then begin transporting the patient to the hospital. A complete head-to-toe survey may be completed while en route to the hospital.

81. **The answer is B.** (AAOS, Scene Size Up and Initial Assessment) Cervical spine injury should always be suspected in an unresponsive trauma patient. Performing the modified jaw thrust while keeping the patient's cervical spine in line will minimize the chance of any further injury to the cervical spine. If blood or secretions are present, they should be cleared by careful suctioning or by carefully rolling the patient onto one side while maintaining cervical spine stabilization.

82. **The answer is D.** (AAOS, Patient Assessment) Rupture of a lung or air passage may cause a leakage of air beneath the skin of the chest. The presence of air bubbles under the surface of the skin will cause a crackling sensation that can be felt on palpation. This is never a normal finding. The presence of this sign should be reported to the hospital staff, because it may indicate a serious underlying injury. This condition may or may not lead to inadequate breathing.

83. **The answer is C.** (Brady, Focused History and Physical Exam—Trauma Patient) An injury to the lung may cause a collection of air or blood in the chest cavity. That will result in decreased breath sounds over that area. This is not a normal finding. A complete airway obstruction will not allow any air movement, and the patient will have no breath sounds. The presence of shock cannot be assessed by listening to breath sounds.

84. **The answer is B.** (AAOS, Patient Assessment) One of the first signs of life-threatening conditions is a change in the level of consciousness. For this reason, the patient's level of consciousness should be assessed frequently. An assessment every 10 minutes is adequate to detect any change that may indicate a serious underlying condition. More frequent assessments can make it easy to miss a gradual change in mental status. Less frequent assessments may allow a serious deterioration to go undetected until it is too late.

85. **The answer is B.** (Mosby, Focused History and Physical Exam—Trauma Patient) Rapid trauma assessment is a quick head-to-toe examination that is used to identify any serious or life-threatening injuries. It may be performed rapidly on the scene or en route to the hospital so as not to delay definitive treatment of a trauma patient. It is not appropriate for all patients but should be done on any patient who has a mechanism of injury that suggests the presence of a severe injury, regardless of age or complaint.

86. **The answer is A.** (Brady, The Initial Assessment) The primary purpose of patient assessment is to identify life-threatening problems so that they may corrected immediately. If a

life-threatening condition is identified, the EMT-Basic should either stabilize it or immediately begin to transport the patient to the hospital. Additional assessments or treatment should not be begun unless the patient can be stabilized.

87. **The answer is B.** (AAOS, Patient Assessment) Ideally, a rapid trauma assessment should be very quick; 1 or 2 minutes should be sufficient to complete the exam. Trauma patients should be transported from the scene within 10 minutes.

88. **The answer is B.** (Mosby, Focused History and Physical Exam—Trauma Patient) If a patient has multiple broken ribs, the chest wall may become unstable. A portion of the chest may then move in the opposite direction from the rest during respiration. This phenomenon is known as *paradoxical respiration*.

89. **The answer is B.** (Brady, the Detailed Physical Exam) The detailed physical examination should not delay transport to the hospital. A rapid primary assessment for life-threatening problems should be conducted immediately. Treatment of life-threatening problems should then be initiated, and transportation begun. The detailed physical examination may be conducted en route to the hospital.

MEDICAL/BEHAVIORAL EMERGENCIES AND OBSTETRICS AND GYNECOLOGY

Directions: Each item below contains four suggested responses. Select the **one best** response to each item.

90. All of the following are medications carried on an EMT-Basic unit EXCEPT

(A) activated charcoal
(B) epinephrine
(C) oral glucose
(D) oxygen

91. As an EMT-Basic, you may assist in administering all of the following medications EXCEPT

(A) epinephrine
(B) an albuterol, metaproterenol, or isoetharine inhaler
(C) digoxin
(D) nitroglycerin

92. An EMT-Basic is able to assist patients administer medications according to four possible routes. These four routes of administration are as follows:

(A) oral, sublingual, subcutaneous, intramuscular
(B) oral, sublingual, inhalational, intramuscular
(C) oral, rectal, cutaneous, intramuscular
(D) oral, subcutaneous, intramuscular, intravenous

93. Which of the following sequences best represents the route that inhaled air takes through the respiratory system?

(A) Larynx, nasopharynx, lung
(B) Trachea, larynx, lung
(C) Nasopharynx, larynx, trachea, bronchus, lung
(D) Bronchus, trachea, nasopharynx, lung

94. Which of the following choices gives the normal resting respiratory rates in breaths per minute for adults, children, and infants?

(A) Adult, 6–10; child, 10–20; infant, 20–30
(B) Adult, 20–30; child, 10–20; infant, 6–10
(C) Adult, 12–20; child, 10–15; infant, 15–20
(D) Adult, 12–20; child, 15–30; infant, 25–50

95. All of the following are signs of respiratory distress EXCEPT

(A) bilateral knee swelling
(B) flaring nostrils, pursed lips, and noisy breathing
(C) increased or decreased respiratory rate
(D) altered mental status, confusion, and anxiety

96. The emergency care of a patient with breathing difficulty may include which of the following?

(A) Administering oxygen
(B) Placing the patient in a position of comfort
(C) Assisting the patient in using a prescribed inhaler
(D) All of the above

97. In assessing a patient with breathing distress, which of the following are signs of inadequate breathing?

(A) A very rapid or very slow respiratory rate
(B) Diminished or absent breath sounds
(C) A diminished level of consciousness accompanied by snoring or gurgling sounds
(D) All of the above

98. In an infant or child, all of the following would be signs of inadequate breathing EXCEPT

(A) retractions of intercostal, supraclavicular, and suprasternal muscles
(B) grunting
(C) unequal pupils
(D) nasal flaring

99. When treating a patient with breathing distress, an EMT-Basic needs medical direction for which of the following treatments?

(A) Administration of oxygen
(B) Use of a prescribed inhaler
(C) Suctioning of the airway
(D) Bag-valve-mask ventilation

100. Which of the following types of patients, when presenting with breathing distress, is most likely to need airway maintenance?

(A) Alert asthmatics
(B) Unconscious patients
(C) Adult patients with fever
(D) Viral influenza patients

101. Asthmatics and patients with known allergies to particular items frequently have a prescribed inhaler. Which of the following is the best classification for the drug in this type of inhaler?

(A) Beta agonist (anticholinergic)
(B) Alpha-agonist (sympathomimetic)
(C) Alpha-agonist (parasympathomimetic)
(D) Beta-agonist (sympathomimetic)

102. All of the following are signs of adequate air exchange EXCEPT

(A) difficulty breathing
(B) sufficient depth of breathing
(C) equal expansion of chest and lungs
(D) equal breath sounds

103. In infants and children, all of the following are signs of difficulty breathing EXCEPT

(A) swollen neck glands
(B) wheezing
(C) use of accessory muscles of respiration
(D) nasal flaring

104. The primary action of beta-agonist metered-dose inhalers is to produce

(A) an increased pulse rate
(B) nasal dilation
(C) sedation
(D) bronchial dilation

105. All the following are contraindications to assisting a patient with the use of a beta-adrenergic agonist metered-dose inhaler EXCEPT

(A) disorientation of the patient
(B) lack of approval by medical direction for providing the assistance
(C) fever with rash
(D) maximum dose already reached

106. Of the following, which is most specifically a sign of upper airway obstruction?

(A) Rapid breathing
(B) Accessory muscle use
(C) Nasal flaring
(D) Stridor

107. For the emergency treatment of breathing difficulty, all of the following measures would be appropriate in infant, children, and adults EXCEPT

(A) putting the patient in a position of comfort
(B) administering oxygen
(C) rapid transport to a hospital
(D) assisting with the administration of a beta-agonist metered-dose inhaler

108. Which of the following sequences best represents the route followed by oxygenated blood after it is pumped from the heart?

(A) Aorta, arteries, arterioles, capillaries
(B) Capillaries, arterioles, arteries, aorta
(C) Arteries, arterioles, capillaries, aorta
(D) Arteries, aorta, capillaries, arterioles

109. All of the following are signs or symptoms of cardiac (heart) disease EXCEPT

(A) chest pain
(B) headache
(C) shortness of breath
(D) abnormal blood pressure and/or pulse

110. The emergency medical care of a patient with chest pain includes all of the following EXCEPT

(A) administration of oxygen
(B) administration of nitroglycerine
(C) administration of epinephrine
(D) provision of basic life support

111. In patients suffering cardiovascular emergencies, which of the following represents the correct positions of comfort?

(A) For difficulty breathing, lying down; for hypotension, sitting up

(B) For either difficulty breathing or hypotension, sitting up

(C) For either difficulty breathing or hypotension, lying down

(D) For difficulty breathing, sitting up; for hypotension, lying down

112. All of the following are indications for assisting a patient with chest pain to administer nitroglycerin EXCEPT that

(A) nitroglycerin is prescribed for the patient

(B) the systolic blood pressure is greater than 100 mm Hg

(C) the patient has palpitations

(D) medical direction authorizes administration

113. All of the following are contra-indications to assisting a chest pain patient self-administer nitroglycerin EXCEPT that

(A) the patient is an infant or child

(B) the patient has a head injury

(C) the patient's systolic blood pressure is less than 100 mm Hg

(D) the patient complains of difficulty breathing

114. When nitroglycerin is used to help relieve a patient's chest pain, it acts by

(A) exerting a tranquilizing effect on the patient

(B) dilating blood vessels

(C) stabilizing the pulse rate

(D) raising the blood pressure

115. Which of the following is an indication for the use of an automated external defibrillator (AED)?

(A) The patient is unresponsive, apneic, and pulseless

(B) The patient has difficulty breathing

(C) The patient has a history of cardiac disease

(D) The patient complains of palpitations

116. Over 600,00 Americans die each year from cardiovascular disease. About how many of these are sudden deaths from out-of-hospital cardiac arrest?

(A) 300,000

(B) 100,000

(C) 500,000

(D) 50,000

117. The American Heart Association has defined the sequence of events that will provide the best chance of survival from sudden, out-of-hospital cardiac arrest, known as the *chain of survival*. All of the following are key links in this chain EXCEPT

(A) early access

(B) early CPR (basic life support)

(C) early defibrillation

(D) early application of military antishock trousers

118. When treating a patient in cardiac arrest, an EMT-Basic may use all of the following airway management maneuvers EXCEPT

(A) suctioning

(B) head-tilt/chin-lift to open the airway

(C) endotracheal intubation

(D) insertion of a nasopharyngeal or oropharyngeal airway

119. Which of the following is the accepted age-or-weight criterion for use of an automated external defibrillator (AED)?

(A) At least 12 years old or at least 90 lb (41 kg)
(B) At least 18 years old or at least 100 lb (45 kg)
(C) At least 10 years old or at least 66 lb (30 kg)
(D) At least 18 years old or at least 90 lb (41 kg)

120. Which of the following interventions on the part of an EMT-Basic has been proved to have the greatest effect on survival in a cardiac arrest patient?

(A) Early defibrillation
(B) Cardiopulmonary resuscitation (CPR)
(C) Assisting with administration of nitroglycerin
(D) Administration of oxygen

121. In providing emergency care to a patient with chest pain and suspected cardiac compromise, an EMT-Basic should routinely institute all of the following interventions EXCEPT

(A) administering high-flow oxygen
(B) attaching the patient to an automated external defibrillator (AED)
(C) placing the patient in a position of comfort
(D) assisting with administration of the patient's nitroglycerin

122. In providing emergency medical care to a patient in cardiac arrest, an EMT-Basic should request advanced life support (ALS) backup (if available in the EMS system). The ALS team would be needed to provide which of the following interventions?

(A) Cardiopulmonary resuscitation
(B) Defibrillation
(C) Endotracheal intubation and administration of intravenous medications
(D) Rapid transport

123. Access to early advanced cardiac life support (ACLS) may be provided in all of the following manners EXCEPT by

(A) an advanced life support (ALS) backup unit
(B) rapid transport to a hospital emergency department
(C) a second EMT-Basic unit
(D) air medical transport

124. Which of the following is the correct way to provide emergency medical care for a patient with chest pain who suddenly goes into cardiac arrest during transport to the hospital?

(A) Stop the unit, defibrillate the patient, provide CPR, and request ALS backup
(B) Provide CPR and rapid transport
(C) Provide high-concentration oxygen, CPR, and rapid transport
(D) Provide CPR, request early hospital notification of incoming cardiac arrest, and begin rapid transport

125. The correct sequence to use in operating the fully automatic AED is which of the following?

(A) Turn on the AED and shock the patient

(B) Hook up two defibrillatory patches to the chest, connect the leads, and turn on the AED

(C) Turn on the AED, then hook up two defibrillatory patches to the chest

(D) Press a button to analyze the rhythm, then attach two defibrillatory patches to the chest

126. The correct sequence to use in operating the semiautomatic AED requires the EMT-Basic to attach the two defibrillatory patches to the patient's chest, connect the leads, turn on the AED, and then

(A) allow the AED to shock the patient automatically

(B) press a button to analyze the rhythm, and proceed as the computer advises

(C) press a button to shock the patient

(D) press a button to analyze the rhythm, and allow the AED to shock the patient automatically

127. Which of the following is the best reason to make sure that a patient is pulseless and apneic before applying an AED?

(A) The AED may advise giving a shock for a patient with a normal sinus rhythm

(B) Use of the AED may worsen cardiac ischemia

(C) The AED may advise giving a shock for a patient in ventricular tachycardia, even though the patient has a pulse and is awake

(D) The process of attaching the AED to the patient may cause a dysrhythmia

128. Which of the following is the reason to avoid using an AED to shock a patient with a pulse with ventricular tachycardia?

(A) Patients with a pulse show no response to defibrillation

(B) Ventricular tachycardia is resistant to defibrillation

(C) AEDs will not advise shock for ventricular tachycardia

(D) Shocking a patient with a pulse may cause ventricular fibrillation or asystole and put the patient in cardiac arrest

129. All of the following situations may lead to shocks being given inappropriately by an AED EXCEPT

(A) ventricular tachycardia in a patient with a pulse
(B) a low charge in the AED's batteries
(C) using the AED on a patient in a moving ambulance
(D) ventricular tachycardia in a patient who is pulseless, apneic, and unconscious

130. Which of the following is the correct reason for not using an AED to shock a patient lying in water or touching any metal?

(A) The shock will be ineffective for defibrillating the patient
(B) Anyone else in contact with the water or metal can get shocked
(C) The AED's batteries will be drained
(D) Multiple shocks will have to be given to defibrillate the patient

131. All of the following statements concerning CPR and the use of the AED are true EXCEPT that

(A) an EMT-Basic who is alone should begin CPR and should await help before using an AED
(B) defibrillation takes priority over CPR in the cardiac arrest patient
(C) the EMT must stop doing CPR before turning on the AED
(D) CPR may be stopped for up to 90 seconds while three consecutive shocks are delivered

132. You are called to the home of a 63-year-old unconscious man. Upon arrival, you find the patient nonresponsive, apneic, and pulseless. Which of the following represents a correct course of action?

(A) CPR should be started before an AED is attached
(B) CPR should be started immediately and stopped for 10-second intervals
(C) CPR should be stopped initially but restarted prior to an AED shock
(D) CPR should be stopped before the AED analyzes the heart rhythm

133. The main advantage of using a fully automatic rather than a semiautomatic AED is that the fully automatic AED

(A) can identify both ventricular and atrial fibrillation
(B) does not require the attachment of leads to the patient
(C) only takes 5 seconds to defibrillate the patient
(D) analyzes the heart rhythm and delivers a shock without action from the operator

134. All of the following are advantages of using a semiautomatic AED EXCEPT that

(A) the computerized rhythm analysis is performed by multiple methods
(B) the device is able to analyze the cardiac rhythm in a moving ambulance
(C) once the rhythm is analyzed, the device advises the operator whether or not to shock
(D) if the device has recommended shocking the patient, the shock is delivered only if the operator presses a button

135. An important disadvantage of using a fully automatic rather than a semi-automatic AED is that

(A) the device is much larger and heavier than a semiautomatic AED

(B) movement of the patient or touching of the patient while the heart rhythm is being analyzed may cause the device to decide that ventricular fibrillation is present even if it is not

(C) the device does not reliably detect ventricular fibrillation when it is present

(D) the device takes much longer to defibrillate a patient than does a semiautomatic AED in experienced hands

136. A fully automatic AED can usually deliver its first shock how soon after it arrives at the patient's side?

(A) 15 seconds

(B) 1 minute

(C) 2 minutes

(D) 5 minutes

137. In operating an AED, which of the following is the correct sequence of actions?

(A) Apply the AED electrodes; establish that the patient is apneic, unconscious, and pulseless; begin CPR

(B) Apply the AED electrodes; turn on the AED; establish that the patient is apneic, unconscious, and pulseless

(C) Establish that the patient is apneic, unconscious, and pulseless; begin CPR; apply the AED electrodes; turn on the AED

(D) Turn on the AED; apply the AED electrodes; begin CPR

138. An EMT-Basic responds to a call and finds a 50-year-old woman in cardiac arrest. The EMT-Basic uses an AED and gives the patient three shocks, as the AED recommends. The patient regains a pulse, but the pulse becomes very rapid. Two paramedics then arrive and determiné from the monitor that the patient has a supraventricular tachycardia. Which of the following features is found on most AEDs and will assist the paramedics in treating the patient?

(A) A manual control module that allows the operator to deliver a shock for rhythms other than the ones for which the AED is programmed to recommend defibrillation

(B) The capacity to defibrillate a patient in less than 1 minute

(C) Adhesive defibrillation pads that permit remote delivery of a shock

(D) The ability to analyze the heart rhythm and recommend whether or not to shock the patient

139. A fact about the AED that makes this device safer for the operator than a manual defibrillator is that the AED

(A) uses less power in delivering a shock

(B) takes more time to set up and deliver a shock

(C) uses "hands-off" adhesive defibrillation pads

(D) can read the heart rhythm and recommend whether or not to shock the patient

140. After attaching a semiautomatic AED to a patient in confirmed cardiac arrest, which of the following is the proper sequence of actions?

(A) Continue CPR, analyze the cardiac rhythm, resume CPR

(B) Stop CPR, make sure all individual are clear of the patient, press the analysis button, and shock the patient if the device advises it

(C) Continue CPR analyze the cardiac rhythm, make sure all individuals are clear of the patient, press the analysis button, and shock the patient if the device advises it

(D) Press the analysis button, continue CPR, and shock the patient if the device advises it

141. A 51-year-old man is in confirmed cardiac arrest. You attach the AED, have the rhythm analyzed, and are advised to shock the patient. You proceed to stop CPR, clear all individuals from the patients, and deliver three consecutive shocks. All of the following statements concerning the further treatment of this patient are true EXCEPT that you should

(A) check for a pulse; if it is absent you should resume CPR for 1 minute

(B) analyze the rhythm after 1 minute of CPR, and, if advised to, administer three additional shocks

(C) after a total of six shocks, check again for a pulse; if it is absent, you should shock three more times for a total of nine shocks

(D) check for a pulse whenever a "No Shock Indicated" message appears

142. A 41-year-old woman in cardiac arrest has just regained a pulse after you administered a second shock (300 J). You check for and maintain an open airway, and transport the patient while maintaining basic life support. However, during transport, the patient again becomes pulseless, apneic, and unresponsive. As an EMT-Basic, you should do which of the following?

(A) Start CPR and continue transport to the emergency department

(B) During transport, analyze the rhythm, and, if advised to, deliver three shocks

(C) Start CPR, call for ACLS backup, and continue transport if the ACLS backup is unavailable

(D) Stop the transport unit, stop CPR, clear all individuals from the patient, analyze the rhythm, and, if advised to, deliver three shocks.

143. When administering two sets of three consecutive shocks as advised by the AED, a pulse check should be performed

(A) six times, once after each shock

(B) twice, after the third and sixth shocks

(C) once, after shock 6

(D) three times, after shocks 2, 4, and 6

144. All of the following are reasons to begin transport of a cardiac-arrest patient EXCEPT that

(A) the patient regains a pulse

(B) two sets of three stacked shocks have been delivered

(C) the AED advises delivering no shock on three consecutive checks

(D) one set of three stacked shocks has been delivered

145. After receiving two sets of three stacked shocks, a cardiac arrest patient remains pulseless, apneic, and unresponsive, and the AED advises shocking the patient. All of the following are treatment options EXCEPT

(A) call for an advanced life support (ALS) unit or air medical transport
(B) contact your medical control to ask if additional shocks should be given
(C) continue to administer AED-advised shocks indefinitely
(D) provide rapid transport, continuing CPR en route

146. You are the only EMT-Basic at the scene of a 73-year-old male chest-pain patient who has just gone into cardiac arrest. After taking body substance isolation precautions, you should proceed with which of the following treatment sequences?

(A) Confirm that the patient is unresponsive, pulseless, and apneic; turn on and attach the AED; perform rhythm analysis, and shock if advised
(B) Start CPR and transport the patient to the emergency department
(C) Start CPR; call for advanced cardiac life support (ACLS) backup; attach the AED; confirm that the patient is unresponsive, pulseless, and apneic; perform rhythm analysis, and shock if advised
(D) Turn on and attach the AED, start CPR, perform rhythm analysis, and shock if advised

147. Which of the following is the American Heart Association's reason for recommending that pulses not be checked during the administration of three consecutive shocks as advised by the AED?

(A) The AED is unable to allow pulse checks
(B) Individuals checking for pulse may be shocked by electricity remaining in the patient
(C) Administration of a series of three stacked shocks results in a better chance of successful defibrillation
(D) The AED is unable to administer one shock at a time

148. An EMT-Basic has administered two sets of three stacked shocks, and the patient remains in cardiac arrest. Which of the following is the best reason for requesting advanced life support (ALS) backup?

(A) ALS units have more powerful manual defibrillators
(B) The manual defibrillators of ALS units are better at analyzing rhythms
(C) ALS units usually are capable of providing faster transport
(D) ALS units deliver early advanced cardiac life support (ACLS), including intubation and intravenous medications

149. All of the following are components of postresuscitation care EXCEPT

(A) resuming CPR if the patient is pulseless and no shock is advised

(B) if the patient is pulseless and shocking is advised, contacting local medical control or following medical control guidelines on what to do

(C) if the patient regains a pulse, transporting without oxygen

(D) requesting an advanced life support (ALS) unit backup

150. Repeated practice in the operation of an automated external defibrillator (AED) is essential for an EMT-Basic to provide a cardiac arrest patient with the best opportunity for survival. At present, this skill is maintained by which of the following?

(A) Repeating the EMT-Basic course every 6 months

(B) Weekly skills-practice sessions with the medical director

(C) Refresher training every 3 months

(D) Mailing in a written exam every month

151. Defibrillators require regular maintenance. On a daily basis, EMT-Basics must complete which of the following?

(A) The defibrillation practice sheet

(B) The AED battery check list

(C) The operator's-shift checklist for automated defibrillators

(D) The American Heart Association's defibrillator rules

152. All of the following are part of the role of the American Heart Association in regulating the use of automated external defibrillators (AEDs), EXCEPT

(A) establishing the chain of survival—early access, early CPR, early defibrillation, early advanced cardiac life support (ACLS)

(B) establishing ACLS standards for ALS backup, including endotracheal intubation and intravenous medications

(C) publishing guidelines and additional information on AEDs

(D) encouraging the use of the AED only after CPR has been performed for 10 minutes

153. All of the following are reasons for providing case review following the use of an AED EXCEPT

(A) to provide EMT-Basics with positive reinforcement or constructive criticism concerning the care given

(B) to review the exact dispatch and response times of each call

(C) to ensure that the AED was used in response to correct indications and that a correct procedure was followed in applying and using the AED

(D) to berate EMT-Basics who applied AEDs to patients who later died

154. The role of the medical director in an EMS system that uses AEDs includes all of the following EXCEPT

(A) overseeing and approving initial training and continuing education in the use of the AED

(B) mechanical repair of each AED

(C) monitoring the quality of care provided with the use of the AED in the EMS system

(D) supervising case review with the EMT-Basics who actually operate the AEDs

155. Which of the following best describes the goal of quality improvement in reviewing each case of AED use?

(A) To provide the best quality of patient care by each EMT-Basic in an EMS system

(B) To discipline EMT-Basics who have unsuccessfully attempted AED resuscitation

(C) To design research articles related to AED resuscitation

(D) To review drug dosing by paramedics

156. An EMT-Basic may prevent the most common cause of the failure of an AED's event recorder by

(A) carrying out a regular program of AED and battery maintenance

(B) reviewing the care of each EMT-Basic patient

(C) attending medical-director case review sessions

(D) performing yearly preventive maintenance on the AEDs

157. All of the following are components of medical direction for the provision of emergency medical care for the chest pain patient EXCEPT

(A) providing verbal or written guidelines for the EMT-Basic assisting a patient in taking prescribed nitroglycerin

(B) providing quality-assurance case review for all aspects of the emergency care of the chest pain patient

(C) trying to provide guidelines for selecting which chest pain patients to treat with new medications

(D) giving instruction regarding potential candidates for blood-clot-dissolving medications and encouraging rapid transport of such patients

158. A 27-year-old woman presents with an altered mental status and a history of diabetes. All of the following are possible patient presentations EXCEPT

(A) confusion due to hypoglycemia

(B) low blood pressure due to hypoglycemia

(C) unconsciousness due to hypoglycemia

(D) hostility and combativeness due to hypoglycemia

159. All of the following are ways to confirm that a patient with an altered mental status is currently taking diabetic medication EXCEPT

(A) taking a history from the patient, the family, a friend, or a coworker

(B) an angry reaction on the part of the patient to all medical history questioning

(C) a medical alert necklace or bracelet

(D) the presence of insulin or oral hypoglycemic medication near the patient, in a purse or briefcase, or in the refrigerator or medicine cabinet

160. A 47-year-old man is acting confused at work. You are called to the scene by coworkers, who confirm that the patient is a known diabetic and that he said he took his insulin early that morning. Which of the following is the proper sequence of steps in providing emergency care to this patient, before administering oral glucose?

(A) Perform, a focused history and physical examination; check the airway, breathing, and circulation; confirm the patient's ability to swallow

(B) Call the patient's physician or pharmacy to check the diabetic medication; check vital signs

(C) Call a family member for the medical/dietary history; call for ALS backup

(D) Administer a test dose of oral glucose to evaluate swallowing ability; check the airway

161. Airway management is of primary concern in managing a patient with altered mental status. All of the following are good reason for this EXCEPT that

(A) airway obstruction from the tongue or oral secretions is common in this situation

(B) airway adjuncts and/or assisted ventilation may be required

(C) the patient's inability to protect the airway is a contraindication to oral glucose administration

(D) patients with altered mental status frequently have anatomically abnormal airways

162. A 23-year-old diabetic man is acting strangely. He has a medical alert badge documenting that he is a diabetic on insulin. After you perform an initial assessment including a focused history, attend to airway management, and repeat the assessment of the airway, breathing, and circulation, medical direction gives you permission to administer glucose. Which of the following are two trade names for forms of oral glucose?

(A) Regular and NPH insulin

(B) Glutose 15 and Insta-glucose

(C) Diabinese and Diabeta

(D) Orinase and Glucophage

163. An EMT-Basic, in administering oral glucose to a diabetic patient with an altered mental status, must make sure that all of the following guidelines are followed EXCEPT that

(A) on-line or off-line medical direction gives approval
(B) the patient is responsive and able to swallow
(C) a full tube of glucose is administered between the patient's cheek and gum
(D) ongoing assessments are performed every 20 minutes

164. All of the following statements concerning the administration of oral glucose to a patient who requires it are true EXCEPT that

(A) oral glucose acts to increase blood glucose (sugar) levels, which will resolve the patient's symptoms
(B) the only contraindication to administering glucose is inability to swallow or unconsciousness
(C) inability to swallow or unconsciousness can lead to aspiration of oral glucose into the lungs
(D) oral glucose administration may cause serious injury to certain alert patients

165. A 23-year-old woman with a known allergy to bee stings has just been stung by a bee. All of the following are possible symptoms in this patient EXCEPT

(A) low blood pressure
(B) itchy skin
(C) tightness in the throat and/or chest
(D) tingling or numbness in the face, mouth, chest, feet, and hands

166. A 14-year-old boy has just eaten a fish dinner in a restaurant. The gravy contained crushed almonds to which he is allergic. As the EMT-Basic assessing this patient, you may find any of the following signs of an allergic reaction EXCEPT

(A) respiratory arrest and coma
(B) hypotension and/or shock
(C) hives, facial swelling, and wheezing
(D) a complaint of headache

167. In patients with severe allergic reactions, progressive respiratory distress may develop. Which of the following best describes the mechanism involved in progressive respiratory distress?

(A) Skin rash and hives
(B) Increased swelling of airway tissues with development of partial or complete airway obstruction
(C) Watery eyes and runny nose
(D) Airway obstruction from a foreign body, associated with wheezing in the chest

168. The emergency care provided by an EMT-Basic to a patient who suffers a severe allergic reaction may include all of the following EXCEPT

(A) administering intravenous medication
(B) administering high-flow oxygen via a non-rebreather mask while completing the initial assessment
(C) rapid transport to the hospital with continuous reassessment of the airway, breathing, and circulation
(D) with the approval of medical direction, assisting the patient to administer a prescribed epinephrine acute-injector (e.g., EpiPen)

169. You are called to assess a 12-year-old girl, who felt sick and swallowed two of her father's amoxicillin antibiotic tablets. The patient admits to having a penicillin allergy and now is complaining of difficulty breathing. Your assessment confirms that she is in respiratory distress with stridor. In beginning to assist the patient in administering her prescribed epinephrine auto-injector, all of the following are correct EXCEPT that

(A) the adult dose of epinephrine delivered by an EpiPen is 0.3 mg, while the infant/child dose of epinephrine delivered is 0.15 mg

(B) two of the prescription devices available to treat severe allergic reactions with self-injectable epinephrine are EpiPen and AnaKit

(C) epinephrine acts rapidly by producing bronchodilation to improve breathing and constricts blood vessels to increase blood pressure

(D) epinephrine injections are contraindicated in patients with heart disease and high blood pressure

170. A 36-year-old woman had just begun working in the garden. She called for an ambulance because of difficulty breathing, hoarseness, hives, and a rapid heartbeat. As the EMT-Basic, you complete your assessment and confirm that the patient is having a severe allergic reaction, manifested by respiratory distress. You receive permission from medical direction to assist the patient in administering her prescribed epinephrine auto-injector. After removing the safety cap from the auto-injector, you wipe the patient's thigh with alcohol. Which of the following is the correct sequence to follow in giving the epinephrine?

(A) Place the auto-injector against the medial part of the thigh, push it firmly against the thigh until the injector activates, and hold it in place until the medication is injected

(B) Place the auto-injector against the middle section of the thigh, push it firmly against the thigh until the injector activates, and hold it in place until the medication is injected

(C) Place the auto-injector against the lateral part of the thigh, push it firmly against the thigh until the injector activates, and hold it in place until the medication is injected

(D) Place the auto-injector against the lateral part of the thigh, push it gently against the thigh until the injector activates, and remove the injector after it is activated.

171. Along with oral ingestion, all of the following are ways that poisons may enter the body EXCEPT

(A) evaporation of liquid toxins contained in a closed bottle
(B) injection by a snake bite, by a sting or bite from an insect, spider, or marine animal, or by a drug needle
(C) inhalation through the airway to the lungs
(D) absorption through the skin

172. Ingested toxins may cause the following signs and symptoms: nausea, vomiting, diarrhea, altered mental status, abdominal pain, chemical burns around the mouth, and certain breath odors. All of the following are possible signs and symptoms of the accompanying type of poisoning EXCEPT

(A) for absorbed toxins—liquid or powder on the patient's skin, burns, redness, itching, irritation of the skin
(B) for injected toxins—diarrhea, abdominal pain, certain breath odors
(C) for inhaled toxins—difficulty breathing, chest pain, cough, hoarseness
(D) for inhaled toxins—dizziness, headache, confusion, seizures, altered mental status

173. An 18-year-old man has been found by a classmate unconscious in his room with an empty, unlabeled pill bottle at his side. The emergency medical care for this unconscious patient with a suspected ingested overdose may include all of the following EXCEPT

(A) checking and maintaining an open airway by inserting an oral or nasal airway, and, if breathing is adequate, administering oxygen
(B) inserting a bite block into the patient's mouth, then attempting to remove any pills, tablets, or fragments from the mouth
(C) consulting medical direction and asking permission to administer activated charcoal
(D) bringing containers, bottles, labels, vomitus, or pill fragments with the patient, as possible evidence of the type of ingestion

174. In administering activated charcoal to a patient with signs and symptoms of an ingested poison, all of the following are true EXCEPT that

(A) for prehospital use, it comes premixed in water and in plastic bottles containing 25 g of activated charcoal
(B) the dose for adults and children is 1 g of activated charcoal per kilogram of body weight
(C) activated charcoal binds poison in the stomach, thereby decreasing absorption of the poison
(D) side effects of the use of activated charcoal are headaches, palpitations, and fever

175. All of the following are trade names for activated charcoal EXCEPT

(A) Insta Char
(B) Actidose
(C) LiquiChar
(D) CharCoal

176. You are called to the scene of a very upset 50-year-old woman who has just been bitten on her right forearm by a reportedly large black spider. The patient complains of feeling weak, dizzy, and nauseous. The site of the bite is red and swollen, and the patient states that it feels like it is burning. All of the following may be part of providing emergency care to a patient suspected to be suffering from injected toxins EXCEPT

(A) determining that the airway is open, administering oxygen, and preparing to suction if the patient vomits
(B) preparing to give a report of the source of injection, the location of the injury, the patient's signs and symptoms, and the treatment given
(C) making all possible attempts to capture the spider as evidence
(D) immobilizing the bitten extremity to slow the circulation of the poison

177. You are dispatched to the home of a depressed 17-year-old boy who had swallowed a bottle of cleaning fluid labeled "poisonous if ingested." After performing a history and physical assessment, you decide that this patient would benefit from the administration of activated charcoal. All of the following are essential in administering activated charcoal EXCEPT

(A) after administering activated charcoal, calling for approval from medical direction
(B) if the patient vomits after swallowing the dose of activated charcoal, repeating the dose once, following orders from medical direction
(C) before giving the patient the liquid activated charcoal to drink, shaking the container to suspend the medication in the liquid
(D) reevaluating the patient after the entire dose of liquid activated charcoal has been swallowed

178. All of the following are correct definitions of ways in which the body loses heat EXCEPT

(A) conduction—transfer of heat from one material to another through direct contact
(B) convection—removal of heat from the stomach by air or water that is swallowed
(C) radiation—heat that the body sends out as electromagnetic waves
(D) evaporation—heat lost when the body perspires or gets wet and the water dries off the skin

179. All of the following are signs and symptoms of hypothermia resulting from exposure to cold EXCEPT

    (A) numbness (reduced or absent ability to feel touch)

    (B) stiff or rigid posture; joint/muscle stiffness or muscle rigidity

    (C) warm abdominal skin temperature

    (D) loss of motor coordination

180. Some of the signs and symptoms in the early stages of hypothermia change in the advanced stages of hypothermia, after prolonged exposure to the cold. All of the following are examples of this EXCEPT that

    (A) shivering is present in early hypothermia, when the core body temperature is above 90°F; shivering decreases and may be absent in severe hypothermia

    (B) in early hypothermia, a patient may be drowsy, uncooperative, and confused, but in late hypothermia the patient becomes stuporous or unconscious

    (C) in early hypothermia, a patient has slow breathing, slow pulse, and low blood pressure, and in later stages, develops a rapid pulse and rapid breathing

    (D) in early hypothermia the skin may be red, but in later stages, the skin is pale to cyanotic

181. You arrive at the scene of a 76-year-old man who is lying in a snow-covered street and complains of feeling cold. Your assessment reveals that the patient is alert and shivering. All of the following would be appropriate emergency care for this hypothermic patient EXCEPT

    (A) removing the patient from the cold street into the ambulance patient compartment and turning up the heat

    (B) not removing wet clothing but putting blankets on the patient over the wet clothing

    (C) wrapping heat packs in towels and placing them in the groin, armpits, neck, and head

    (D) administering warmed and humidified oxygen if available

182. You are called to the scene of an 80-year-old man who was found in a very cold outside garage. Your assessment reveals a very confused, disoriented patient lying on an ice-cold cement floor. His abdominal skin is very cold to the touch. All of the following are part of the emergency care indicated for this patient EXCEPT

    (A) covering him with warm blankets

    (B) administering high-flow oxygen

    (C) placing heat packs in towels in the groin, armpits, neck, and head

    (D) turning up the heat in the patient compartment of the ambulance

183. You have been dispatched to a cardiac arrest in the backyard of a home. Upon arrival, you find a 50-year-old woman who was reported to having been drinking heavily the night before and was found lying in her backyard on the ground, on a truly freezing winter morning. The patient is unresponsive, has very cold abdominal skin, is not breathing, and does not have a pulse. The emergency care of this patient would include all of the following EXCEPT

(A) opening and maintaining an airway
(B) administering 100% oxygen
(C) contacting medical control about the use of an automated external defibrillator (AED)
(D) checking for a pulse for 10 seconds and, if no pulse is found, beginning CPR

184. The following are all signs and symptoms of hyperthermia caused by exposure to heat, EXCEPT

(A) frequent urination
(B) muscle cramps
(C) moist, pale, cool, or normal skin
(D) altered mental status

185. You are dispatched on a hot summer day to an 85-year-old man who is weak and confused. Upon entering his apartment, you immediately feel intensely hot. The patient is lying on this bed, responsive, with a winter coat on, and all of the windows closed. The patient's skin feels moist and cool and appears pale. The emergency care for this patient includes all of the following EXCEPT

(A) immediately moving the patient to a cool area
(B) removing his winter coat and loosening or removing other clothing
(C) allowing the patient to sit upright in the stretcher
(D) cooling the patient by fanning

186. You are dispatched to an unresponsive patient in the basement of an old hotel. Upon arrival, you find a 68-year-old man lying in a very hot boiler room, barely responsive to painful stimuli. The skin feels hot and dry. The emergency care of this patient should include all of the following EXCEPT

(A) optional administration of oxygen
(B) removing clothing, applying cold packs to the neck, groin, and armpits, and keeping the skin wet by applying water with a sponge or wet towels
(C) removing the patient to a cool environment and fanning aggressively
(D) immediate transport

187. Which of the following sets of findings indicates the most serious need for emergency care for heat exposure?

(A) Weakness and hot, dry skin

(B) Muscle cramps and moist, pale, cool skin

(C) Exhaustion and dizziness with moist, pale skin that is normal in temperature

(D) A weak pulse and rapid breathing with moist, pale, cool skin

188. All of the following findings are common in water-related emergencies EXCEPT

(A) airway obstruction

(B) head and neck injuries

(C) hyperthermia

(D) substance abuse

189. You are dispatched to a beach where a 17-year-old has been pulled out of the ocean in a near-drowning incident. As you drive to the scene you think of the possible complications of near-drowning incidents. All of the following are complications of near-drowning EXCEPT

(A) spinal injuries

(B) airway obstruction

(C) gastric distention, which may lead to vomiting with aspiration into the lungs

(D) skin rash

190. You are dispatched to a 17-year-old girl who was "stung by a bee." Upon arrival, you find the patient crying and pointing to a stinger still in place in her right arm. All of the following would be part of emergency care of a patient with a bite or sting EXCEPT

(A) confirming adequate airway, breathing, and circulation

(B) removing jewelry from the injured area before swelling occurs

(C) if the injury is to an extremity, positioning the bite or sting site above the level of the heart

(D) observing the patient closely for any signs and symptoms of an allergic reaction

191. Which of the following is the correct way to remove a stinger from the skin of a sting victim?

(A) Carefully use fine tweezers to remove the stinger intact

(B) Scrape out the stinger with the edge of a piece of cardboard, a butter knife, or a plastic card (credit card)

(C) With gloved fingers, squeeze the base of the stinger until the stinger falls out

(D) Rub the stinger site vigorously against a hard surface until the stinger falls out

192. Which of the following is the best definition of a behavioral emergency?

    (A) When a patient's behavior is not typical for the situation; is unacceptable or intolerable to the patient, the patient's family, or the community; or may harm the patient or others

    (B) When a patient's behavior would be judged as rude by a complete stranger

    (C) When the patient calmly expresses political views which are different than those of his family and/or friends

    (D) When a child's behavior is judged to be selfish, fresh, or stubborn

193. You are dispatched to an emotionally disturbed 51-year-old person, in the middle of the main street in your town. As you are driving to the scene you reflect on general factors that may result in an alteration of a patient's behavior. All of the following are possible physical causes of altered behavior EXCEPT

    (A) hypoglycemia, drugs, alcohol, poisoning

    (B) hypothermia, hyperthermia, hypoxia

    (C) head trauma, stroke (cerebrovascular accident or transient ischemic attack)

    (D) skin rash, hair loss

194. All of the following are possible reasons for psychological crisis EXCEPT

    (A) depression

    (B) paranoid psychosis

    (C) mania

    (D) insomnia

195. You are dispatched to a family disturbance, yet upon your arrival you find a 22-year-old girl quietly sitting in a chair in the kitchen. The family is in a heated argument over "why this patient may want to kill herself." All of the following are personal characteristics which suggest that the patient may be at risk for suicide EXCEPT

    (A) a family history of suicide by the patient's adopted parents

    (B) the patient recently lost a job, got divorced, or experienced the death of a family member or close friend

    (C) at the scene, there is an unusual gathering of dangerous articles (pills, guns, etc.)

    (D) the patient has made previous attempts and/or present threats of suicide

196. In dealing with a patient with a behavioral emergency, all of the following statements are true EXCEPT that

    (A) patients who, in your judgment, are a threat to themselves or others may be transported after medical direction is contacted

    (B) when a patient with a behavioral emergency refuses your treatment, you should contact law enforcement for assistance

    (C) in restraining a patient for emergency transport, it is acceptable to place a gag in the patient's mouth

    (D) in attempting to treat patients without consent, it is important to know both your state law and local medical protocol concerning this topic

197. You respond to a call and find an open door to a third-floor apartment. You immediately see a 53-year-old man sitting in a chair. He appears very upset, fists clenched, staring out with a large knife next to him. Which of the following is the correct way to proceed?

(A) Directly approach the patient while your partner makes a quick move for the knife

(B) Do not enter the apartment; call for law enforcement assistance and await their arrival

(C) Enter the apartment and allow the patient to position himself between you and the door

(D) Try to verbally provoke the patient into displaying his hostile thoughts or actions

198. All of the following are signs that a patient is at risk for violent behavior EXCEPT that the patient

(A) has clenched fists

(B) is standing or moving toward the EMT

(C) is holding a potentially dangerous object

(D) is calmly explaining his problems

199. In approaching the patient with a behavioral emergency, it is essential to try to calm the patient. The following are all methods used to try to calm the patient EXCEPT

(A) asking questions in a calm, reassuring manner and showing that you are listening by repeating part of the patient's answers

(B) speaking with the patient in a calm, honest, reassuring manner, not arguing, threatening or showing any indication of using force

(C) trying to work fast and quickly; encouraging the patient to co-operate and go the hospital immediately

(D) seeking the help of trusted family members and/or friends to calm the patient

200. All of the following are predelivery emergencies EXCEPT

(A) retained placenta

(B) miscarriage

(C) seizures

(D) vaginal bleeding

201. In the pregnant female label the following anatomic structures: uterus, vagina, fetus, placenta, umbilical cord, amniotic sac, perineum, cervix, bladder, and anus.

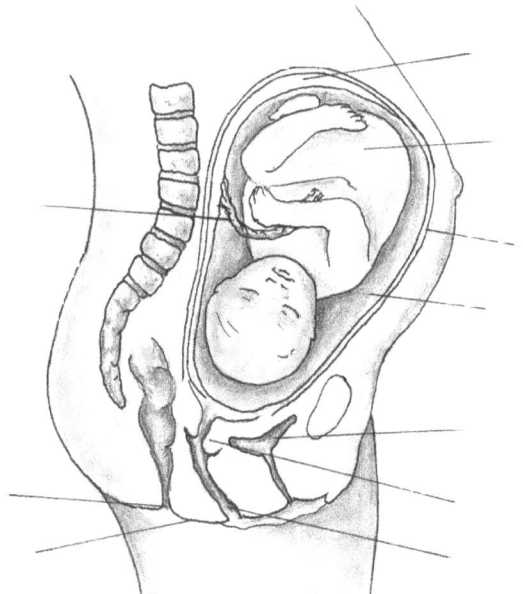

202. The obstetrics (OB) kit contains supplies that are needed to assist with the delivery of an infant. All of the following choices represent items in this kit, with correct descriptions of their function EXCEPT which one?

(A) Hemostats or cord clamps—used to clamp the umbilical cord

(B) Surgical scissors or scalpel (surgical knife)—used to cut the umbilical cord

(C) Umbilical tape or sterilized cord—used to tie the umbilical cord

(D) Sterile gloves—to be worn only after the delivery to care for the newborn infant

203. You are dispatched to the scene of a 19-year-old woman who is "having a miscarriage." Upon arrival, the patient confirms that she is 6 weeks pregnant and began to have heavy vaginal bleeding about an hour ago. All of the following are parts of emergency care rendered to a patient having a miscarriage EXCEPT

(A) with the use of body substance isolation precautions, performing an initial assessment, with baseline measurement of vital signs to aid in the recognition of signs of shock

(B) gently covering the vagina with sterile pads, to control bleeding

(C) gently pulling out any tissue present in the vagina

(D) collecting any tissue that passes out of the vagina and bringing it to the hospital

204. You arrive at the scene of a 27-year-old woman who is 9 months pregnant and states that she has been having contractions for over 12 hours. All of the following are indications of an imminent delivery EXCEPT that

(A) the uterine contractions are 2 to 3 minutes apart and last for 45 to 60 seconds

(B) on inspection, the baby is crowning

(C) the mother feels tingling in her lower legs

(D) the mother feels the urge to push the baby out

205. You are dispatched to a 31-year-old woman who is 8 months pregnant and is complaining of heavy vaginal bleeding. Upon arrival, you find that the patient is not in labor, having not experienced any uterine contractions. She has saved eight sanitary napkins, which are soaked in blood, and her blood pressure is 74/50. The emergency care of this pregnant patient with vaginal bleeding should include which of the following?

(A) Remain at the patient's home until labor begins and deliver the infant

(B) Encourage the patient to lie on her back

(C) Before beginning to care for this patient, carefully follow body substance isolation techniques and even double-glove

(D) Before transport and after arriving at the hospital, discard all bloodied sanitary napkins before bringing the patient inside the emergency department

206. You arrive at the home of a 36-year-old pregnant woman. Her family states that they found her unconscious in bed only 10 minutes ago. The patient is 8 months pregnant, with high blood pressure and gradually increasing swelling of the face, hand, and feet. In your presence, the patient has a grand mal tonic-clonic seizure. The emergency care of this patient should include all of the following EXCEPT

(A) opening and maintaining the airway

(B) not suctioning the patient under any circumstances

(C) administering high-concentration oxygen

(D) handling gently and transporting her on her left side

207. You are dispatched to the scene of a motor vehicle accident. One of the victims is a 26-year-old woman who is 7½ months pregnant. She was in the driver's seat and hit her head on the dashboard; she is complaining of neck and back pain. Which of the following is uniquely a part of the emergency care of this traumatic predelivery emergency?

(A) Administering high-concentration oxygen

(B) Providing emotional support

(C) Immobilizing the patient on a spine board, then tipping the board and patient, as a unit, to the left

(D) Being prepared to suction as needed

208. All of the following are steps in the predelivery preparation for an imminent delivery EXCEPT

(A) taking body substance isolation precautions, including use of gowns, caps, face masks, eye protection, and sterile gloves

(B) placing the mother on a bed, ambulance stretcher, or sturdy table, with the buttocks elevated by blankets or a pillow and the knees drawn up and spread apart

(C) positioning all assistants, including the father and the mother's personal assistant behind you, so that the mother's head is alone and clear

(D) removing any of the mother's underclothing that obstructs your view of the vagina

209. All of the following are steps in assisting the mother in the delivery of her infant EXCEPT

(A) positioning your gloved hands at the vaginal opening as the baby's head appears

(B) when the infant's head appears, applying gentle pressure to prevent an explosive delivery

(C) if the amniotic sac has not broken, leave it alone

(D) as the baby's head is delivered, checking to see if the umbilical cord is wrapped around the baby's neck

210. In preparing a pregnant female for an imminent delivery, all of the following are correct placements for sheets or towels EXCEPT

(A) one under the head
(B) one under the buttocks
(C) one over each thigh
(D) one over the abdomen

211. You are assisting a 30-year-old mother in delivering an infant. The baby's head has just delivered, and you find that the umbilical cord is wrapped around the baby's neck. Which of the following is the correct initial approach to this problem?

(A) Gently continuing the delivery with close observation of the umbilical cord
(B) Immediately trying to force the baby's head back into the vagina, so that the cord may come free of the baby's neck
(C) Trying to place two fingers under the cord at the back of the baby's neck and then trying to bring the cord forward over the baby's upper shoulder and head
(D) Immediately clamping the cord in two places, then cutting the cord between the two clamps, and then gently unwrapping the ends of the cord from around the baby's neck and proceeding with the delivery

212. You are dispatched to an apartment to assist a mother delivering her baby. As you arrive you see the baby's head crowning at the vaginal opening. You prepare for the delivery by instituting body substance isolation precautions, then performing a predelivery history and physical assessment, and then placing sterile towels and barriers. Which of the following is the correct way to care for the baby as the head delivers?

(A) Gently support the head with a gloved hand, wipe the baby's mouth and nose, and then suction the mouth and nose with a bulb syringe
(B) Put heavy traction on the head to expedite the delivery of the remainder of the body
(C) Leave the head alone and deal with the cleaning of blood and mucus; suction the baby's mouth and nose after the entire delivery is completed
(D) With both gloved hands, support the head and prevent any rotation; withhold suctioning until the full delivery is over

213. After a normal vaginal delivery, the correct time to clamp and cut the umbilical cord is

(A) 15 to 20 minutes after the delivery
(B) 5 to 10 minutes after the delivery
(C) after the baby has been bathed and the placenta has been delivered
(D) after the baby is confirmed to be breathing on its own and palpation of the cord reveals no pulsations

214. All of the following are steps to be taken in cutting the umbilical cord EXCEPT

(A) using sterile clamps or umbilical tape from the obstetrics kit
(B) placing a clamp 8 to 10 inches from the baby and a second clamp 6 to 8 inches from the baby (this is about four fingers' width from the baby)
(C) cutting the cord about 14 inches from the baby, beyond the two clamps
(D) examining the cut fetal end of the cord for bleeding, and if bleeding continues, applying another clamp or umbilical tape tie as close to the original clamp or tie as possible

215. You have just assisted a 30-year-old mother in a normal vaginal delivery of a healthy baby. You have clamped and cut the umbilical cord without a problem. All of the following are true concerning the delivery of the placenta EXCEPT that

(A) placental delivery usually occurs 60 to 120 minutes after delivery
(B) placental delivery is usually accompanied by a brief return of labor pains, which had stopped when the baby was born
(C) it is important to save all after-birth tissues in a container, as the attending physician will want to exam them at the hospital for completeness
(D) any afterbirth tissues that remain in the mother after delivery create a serious threat for infection and prolonged bleeding to the mother

216. After assisting a mother in delivering a normal-appearing infant, you expect the child to begin breathing on its own within

(A) 45 to 60 seconds
(B) 1 to 1.5 minutes
(C) a few seconds to 30 seconds
(D) 2 to 3 minutes

217. After assisting the mother in a normal delivery of a healthy infant, all of the following are steps in providing emergency medical care to the mother after the delivery EXCEPT

(A) providing oxygen and immediate transport if the placenta has not delivered after 30 minutes, or if 250 mL of bleeding occurs prior to delivery of the placenta, or if significant bleeding occurs after the placenta is delivered
(B) after the placenta is delivered, if there is significant bleeding, digitally examining the vagina
(C) placing the baby at the mother's breast and allowing it to nurse
(D) placing a sterile pad or sanitary napkin over the vagina and lowering the mother's legs

218. After assisting a mother in a normal vaginal delivery, if the newborn infant does not begin breathing, all of the following techniques should be used EXCEPT

(A) gentle, vigorous rubbing of the baby's back
(B) flicking the soles of the baby's feet
(C) holding the baby upside down and slapping the buttocks
(D) if the above fails, bag-valve-mask ventilations beginning at a rate of 40 to 60 per minute

219. In evaluating the heart rate of a non-breathing newborn as part of neonatal resuscitation, all of the following are true EXCEPT that

(A) if the baby's heart rate is below 100 beats per minute, you should continue artificial ventilations at 60 per minute for another 30 seconds

(B) if, 30 seconds after the first heart rate assessment, the baby's heart rate is still below 80 beats per minute, you should start cardiac chest compressions according to newborn CPR standards

(C) if, upon any reassessment of the baby, the baby's heart rate is above 100 beats per minute and the baby is breathing spontaneously, you should stop artificial ventilations and compressions and administer free-flow oxygen

(D) free-flow oxygen is administered by placing oxygen tubing directly inside the baby's mouth

220. You are in the process of assisting a mother in delivering a baby when you notice that the infant is not breathing. You have tried to stimulate the baby, have flicked the baby's heels, and have begun to assist ventilations with a bag-valve-mask at 40 to 60 breaths per minute. Which of the following should be your next step?

(A) Evaluate the infant's heart rate

(B) Attempt to again suction the airway

(C) Try again to stimulate the child with back rubs and heel flicks

(D) Call medical control for advice

221. You are called to the scene to assist a 30-year-old mother in delivering an infant. As the mother begins to push, you notice that the buttocks are presenting first. All of the following are steps in providing emergency care for a breech delivery EXCEPT

(A) providing the mother with high-concentration oxygen

(B) firmly pulling on the legs (for a legs-first breech delivery)

(C) placing the mother in a head-down position with an elevated pelvis

(D) initiating rapid transport

222. You are assisting a mother with either a legs-first or buttocks-first breech delivery, and the entire body has been delivered. However, the head does not deliver right away. All the following are part of the actions taken to attempt to prevent the baby from suffocating EXCEPT

(A) placing a gloved hand into the vagina with your palm facing the baby's face

(B) making a V with your index and middle fingers on each side of the baby's face

(C) trying to push the vaginal wall away from the baby's face until the head is delivered

(D) if all else fails, pulling strongly on the trunk or legs of the infant

223. You are assisting a 26-year-old mother with her first delivery. Upon inspection, as the mother begins to push, you notice that the first part to deliver is the umbilical cord (known as a prolapsed cord). The reason this situation is a true emergency is because the prolapsed cord

(A) is prone to becoming infected
(B) will cause recurrent vomiting by the baby
(C) is squeezed between the baby's head and the vaginal wall, which may pinch the cord and interrupt the oxygen supply to the baby
(D) may be damaged unless immediately reinserted into the vagina

224. You respond to a 27-year-old woman who is in active labor. Upon assessing the patient, you note that the infant's head is crowning with each contraction. You assist the mother with the delivery of a healthy baby boy. Which of the following is a sign that this mother is about to deliver an additional baby (or babies)?

(A) The first baby is large
(B) The mother's abdomen remains fairly large after the delivery
(C) After 2 to 3 hours, uterine contractions begin again
(D) If there is a second baby, the delivery will occur before the delivery of the first baby's placenta

225. All of the following are true concerning the presence of meconium (fetal stool) in the amniotic fluid EXCEPT that

(A) the color of meconium-stained amniotic fluid is usually reddish-tan
(B) the presence of meconium in the amniotic fluid usually is a sign of fetal distress before or during labor
(C) if the baby aspirates meconium (breathes it into the lungs), serious breathing problems may develop
(D) if you see meconium-stained amniotic fluid, it is essential to suction the mouth and oropharynx before stimulating the baby

226. You respond to the home of a 30-year-old woman who is in the process of delivering a premature infant (6 months after conception). In providing emergency medical care to a premature infant, all of the following are true EXCEPT that you should

(A) keep the infant warm and wrapped in a blanket
(B) suction as needed
(C) if the umbilical cord is bleeding, remove the clamp and only compress the cord with your fingers
(D) administer free-flow oxygen to the infant

227. The emergency care of a patient with a gynecologic emergency that is manifested by shock from severe vaginal bleeding includes all of the following EXCEPT

(A) packing the vagina with sterile dressings
(B) administering oxygen
(C) observing body substance isolation precautions
(D) documenting vital signs

228. You have been dispatched to a college dormitory, where you find a 19-year-old woman who claims that she has just been raped. Which of the following is an important part of delivering emergency care to a sexual assault victim?

(A) Even if the patient is not bleeding, immediately examining the genital area
(B) Encouraging the patient to shower and use the bathroom prior to transport
(C) Using restraints, if needed, to force transport of the sexual assault victim to the hospital
(D) Soothing and calming the patient during transport to the hospital

MEDICAL/BEHAVIORAL EMERGENCIES AND OBSTETRICS AND GYNECOLOGY

A N S W E R S

90. The answer is B. (AAOS, General Pharmacology) All EMT-Basic units carry activated charcoal, oral glucose, and oxygen. Epinephrine is a medication, but, while an EMT-Basic may assist a patient in administering it by medical control, it is not carried on the unit.

91. The answer is C. (AAOS, General Pharmacology) An EMT-Basic may assist in administering epinephrine, nitroglycerine, and metered-dose inhalers containing an oral beta-agonist (albuterol, metaproterenol, or isoetharine). The medication must be prescribed by a physician, and the EMT-Basic must be authorized by medical control to assist in administering it. Digoxin is a common cardiac medication used for treatment of congestive heart failure and certain arrhythmias. It is not approved for assisted administration by an EMT-Basic.

92. The answer is B. (Mosby, General Pharmacology) The four approved routes of administration are oral, sublingual, inhalational, and intramuscular. Other routes of administration that are not approved for EMT-Basic assistance are intravenous, subcutaneous (injections under the skin), cutaneous (e.g., applying nitroglycerin paste to a patient's skin), and rectal (e.g., valium given per rectum to a child who is having seizures and does not have intravenous access). EMT-paramedics usually may use all of the above routes of administration.

93. The answer is C. (Mosby, Respiratory Emergencies) Inhaled air passes from the pharynx (nasopharynx and oropharynx) via the larynx (voice box) into the trachea. From there, it passes down the right and left mainstem bronchi into the lungs.

94. The answer is D. (Mosby, Respiratory Emergencies) The normal range of respiratory rates in breaths per minute are: adult, 12–20; child, 15–30; infant, 25–50.

95. The answer is A. (Brady, Respiratory Emergencies) Signs of respiratory distress include all the ones listed in B, C, and D, as well as increased or decreased pulse rate, changes in breathing rhythm, inability to speak sentences, use of accessory muscles for breathing, coughing, patient positioning, unusual anatomy, and unequal breath sounds. Bilateral knee swelling is not a sign of respiratory distress.

96. **The answer is D.** (Brady, Respiratory Emergencies) The emergency care of a patient with breathing difficulty may include all of the measures listed in the choices, provided the patient has adequate breathing. If the patient has inadequate breathing, then the emergency care that should be given is that for the patient with breathing distress.

97. **The answer is D.** (Mosby, Respiratory Emergencies) Signs of inadequate breathing include all the ones listed in the question choices, as well as shortness of breath, restlessness, a preference for an upright sitting position, an increased pulse rate (in infants and children, an increased or decreased pulse rate), skin color changes (cyanosis, pallor, flushing), retractions or use of accessory muscles, inability to speak, coughing, and an irregular breathing rhythm.

98. **The answer is C.** (Mosby, Respiratory Emergencies) Signs of inadequate breathing in infants and children include the ones listed in A, B, and D, as well as a seesaw pattern of breathing, and noisy breathing. The signs typical for adults may also be present (see the answer and explanation to the preceding question). Unequal pupils are not related to inadequate breathing.

99. **The answer is B.** (Mosby, Respiratory Emergencies) In treating patients in breathing distress, administering oxygen, placing the patient in the position of comfort, suctioning the airway, performing artificial ventilation (mouth-to-mask, bag-valve-mask, oxygen-powered device) are all basic EMT-Basic modalities and can be performed at the EMT-Basic's discretion. However, to assist a patient in using a prescribed inhaler, the EMT-Basic must have specific medical direction, either obtained by speaking to a physician by telephone/radio or specified by written protocols or standing orders.

100. **The answer is B.** (AAOS, Respiratory Emergencies) While attention to the airway is important in all patients suffering from breathing distress, it is particularly important in unconscious patients. The unconscious patient is unable to protect the airway, which can easily become occluded by the tongue, mucus, foreign bodies, dentures, or regurgitated stomach contents.

101. **The answer is D.** (AAOS, Respiratory Emergencies) Beta-agonist agents, when inhaled, produce actions like the beta effects of epinephrine. Epinephrine is a natural hormone secreted by the sympathetic nervous system (a sympathomimetic). When inhaled, beta agonists produce dilation of narrowed bronchial tubes (known as bronchodilation), which results in easier air exchange and may ease breathing in these patients.

102. **The answer is A.** (Mosby, Respiratory Emergencies) Signs of adequate air exchange are an adequate depth of breathing (adequate *tidal volume*), equal chest and lung expansion, equal

breath sounds, and effortless breathing with a normal respiratory rate (adult, 12 to 20 breaths per minute; child, 15 to 30 breaths per minute; and infant, 25 to 50 breaths per minute).

103. **The answer is A.** (AAOS, Respiratory Emergencies) In infants and children, signs of difficulty breathing are wheezing (which represents difficulty in exhaling), use of accessory muscles (such as supraclavicular, suprasternal, and intercostal muscles), nasal flaring, see-saw respirations (due to alternating contractions of chest and abdominal muscles), an increased respiratory rate (tachypnea), and a decreased respiratory rate (bradypnea). Swollen neck glands are usually a sign of a throat infection, not difficulty breathing.

104. **The answer is D.** (AAOS, Respiratory Emergencies) The main action of beta-agonist metered-dose inhalers is to elicit bronchial dilation. The drug causes the smooth muscle in the walls of the bronchial tubes to relax, allowing the bronchial tubes to dilate. The result is easier inhalation and exhalation. Beta-agonists can produce an increased pulse rate as a side effect. Nasal dilation and sedation are not effects of these drugs.

105. **The answer is C.** (Mosby, Respiratory Emergencies) Another contraindication to the use of a beta-agonist-metered-dose inhaler would be if the inhaler were prescribed for another person. Fever with rash is often caused by a viral infection. Viral infections frequently trigger attacks of breathing difficulty in asthmatics.

106. **The answer is D.** (Mosby, Respiratory Emergencies) With upper or lower airway obstruction, a patient may present with rapid breathing, accessory muscle use, and nasal flaring. However, *stridor*—defined as a harsh sound heard during breathing (usually inhalation)—specifically indicates upper airway obstruction. It may occur in adults but is much more common in infants and children. The treatment is gentle administration of oxygen, placing the patient in a position of comfort (for infants and children, being held by a parent), and constant reassessment.

107. **The answer is D.** (Mosby, Respiratory Emergencies) In adults and many children over the age of 6 or 7 years, all of the measures listed in the question choices are appropriate. Infants and most children under the age of 6 or 7 lack the coordination necessary to use inhalers correctly.

108. **The answer is A.** (AAOS, Cardiac Emergencies) The heart pumps oxygenated blood into the aorta, which distributes it to the arteries, which divide into arterioles, which divide into tiny capillaries. Capillaries deliver oxygen and nutrients to the body cells and connect to venules. The venules return the deoxygenated blood and waste to the veins, which deliver it to the superior and inferior venae cavae (draining the upper and lower body, respectively), which empty directly into the heart.

109. **The answer is B.** (AAOS, Cardiac Emergencies) The *symptoms* (patient's complaints) of heart disease are chest pains with possible radiation to one or both arms, the neck, jaw, or upper back; sweating; shortness of breath; anxiety or a feeling of impending doom; palpitations (felt irregularity of the heartbeat); weakness; nausea or vomiting; and epigastric abdominal pain or indigestion. The *signs* (assessment findings) are abnormal and irregular pulse, abnormal blood pressure, difficulty breathing, and the general appearance of an anxious, sweating, pale, cyanotic, patient in acute distress. A patient suffering heart disease may experience many or few of these signs and symptoms.

110. **The answer is C.** (Mosby, Cardiovascular Emergencies) Epinephrine is a drug that is used in the treatment of both severe allergic reactions and cardiac emergencies. An EMT-Basic may help to administer it for the former indication, but not for the latter. The emergency medical care of the patient with chest pain includes administration of high-flow oxygen (15 liters per minute) by a non-rebreather mask, administration of nitroglycerine if it is prescribed for the patient and if administration is approved by medical control, placing the patient in a position of comfort, and providing basic life support, if necessary.

111. **The answer is D.** (Brady, Cardiac Emergencies) Patients with difficulty breathing from any cause usually prefer the sitting-up position. Hypotensive patients (systolic blood pressure less than 90 mm Hg) usually feel better lying down. The latter position provides better blood flow to the brain.

112. **The answer is C.** (Brady, Cardiac Emergencies) The indications for assisting a patient to administer nitroglycerin are that the patient has chest pain and a history of cardiac problems, that nitroglycerin has been prescribed for the patient, that systolic blood pressure exceeds 100 mm Hg, and that medical direction authorizes this measure. The patient must also have nitroglycerin on hand. Palpitations (a feeling of a fast, strong, or irregular heartbeat) may or may not be present in such a patient but is not an indication for nitroglycerin administration.

113. **The answer is D.** (Mosby, Cardiovascular Emergencies) Contraindications to assisting a patient to administer nitroglycerin are that the patient is an infant or child, that the patient has a head injury or is not mentally alert, that the patient's systolic blood pressure is less than 100 mm Hg, that the patient has already taken the maximum prescribed dose, and that the patient either does not have a prescription for nitroglycerin or does not have the drug on hand. While many patients with chest pain and a history of cardiac disease also complain of difficulty breathing, that is neither an indication nor a contraindication to assisting with the administration of nitroglycerin.

114. **The answer is B.** (Brady, Cardiac Emergencies) Nitroglycerin acts by dilating blood vessels. The result is that more blood stays in the veins of the body (venous pooling), so there is less blood coming back to the heart. With less blood to pump, the heart does not have to work as hard. Nitroglycerin does not have a tranquilizing effect. Its side effects are headache, a burning sensation on or under the tongue, lowered blood pressure, and changes in pulse rate.

115. The answer is A. (Brady, Cardiac Emergencies) The only indication for the use of an automated external defibrillator (AED) is that the patient is in cardiac arrest—unresponsive, apneic (not breathing), and pulseless. The two shockable rhythms are ventricular fibrillation and ventricular tachycardia. Use of this device is not appropriate for a patient who is awake and alert with ventricular tachycardia (and who thus is not in cardiac arrest and not pulseless).

116. The answer is A. (Brady, Cardiac Emergencies) Over 600,000 Americans dies of cardiovascular disease each year. This number includes deaths from heart attacks, heart failure, strokes, ruptured aneurysms, poor peripheral circulation, etc. Half of these deaths occur outside the hospital as out-of-hospital cardiac arrests. This fact truly emphasizes the importance of the chain of survival, early access, early cardiopulmonary resuscitation, early defibrillation, and early advanced cardiac life support.

117. The answer is D. (AAOS, Cardiac Emergencies) The chain of survival includes early access to the EMS system, early cardiopulmonary resuscitation (CPR), early defibrillation, and early advanced cardiac life support (ACLS), including intubation and intravenous medications. Early application of military antishock trousers is not a part of this chain.

118. The answer is C. (Mosby, Cardiovascular Emergencies) While early defibrillation is of primary importance in resuscitating a patient in cardiac arrest, early cardiopulmonary resuscitation (CPR) is another key link in the chain of survival. Early CPR can only be performed with an airway that is correctly kept open and clear. Endotracheal intubation is an advanced airway management maneuver, not performed by EMT-Basics.

119. The answer is A. (Mosby, Cardiovascular Emergencies) The accepted criterion for use of an AED is that the patient be at least 12 years old or at least 90 lb (41 kg) in weight. If the patient is younger or lighter than this, an EMT-Basic must consult medical direction or follow local protocol regarding the use of an AED.

120. The answer is A. (Mosby, Cardiovascular Emergencies) The American Heart Association's text on advanced cardiac life support states that early defibrillation is the only intervention that has been proved to improve the survival of a cardiac arrest patient. CPR and oxygen administration are important in the treatment of patients in cardiac arrest. While assisting with the administration of nitroglycerin is an important part of emergency medical care in a patient with chest pain, it is not a part of the treatment of cardiac arrest.

121. The answer is B. (Brady, Cardiac Emergencies) Emergency medical care for a patient with chest pain and cardiac compromise does include administering high-flow oxygen, placing the patient in position of comfort, assisting with administration of the patient's nitroglycerin, and providing basic life support (CPR) if necessary. However, most patients with chest pain are not having a heart attack, and many have no heart problem at all. Therefore, attaching an AED to the patient would be inappropriate.

122. The answer is C. (AAOS, Cardiac Emergencies) Early advanced cardiac life support (ACLS) is the fourth and final link in the chain of survival for the cardiac arrest patient. The advanced life support (ALS) team is capable of inserting an endotracheal tube to provide the best airway to ventilate the patient and can also administer intravenous medications to assist in resuscitating the patient. The EMT-Basic team is able to provide CPR, defibrillation with an automated external defibrillator, and rapid transport.

123. The answer is C. (AAOS, Cardiac Emergencies) Choices A, B, and D all represent ways in which early ACLS may be provided for the cardiac arrest patient, depending on the EMS system. Neither a first nor a second EMT-Basic unit is certified to administer ACLS interventions.

124. The answer is A. (Mosby, Cardiovascular Emergencies) The American Heart Association has determined that early defibrillation is the one intervention proved to improve cardiac arrest survival. Therefore, should a patient go into cardiac arrest during transport, the EMT-Basic should stop the unit, defibrillate, provide CPR, and request advanced life support (ALS) backup.

125. The answer is B. (Mosby, Cardiovascular Emergencies) There are two types of automatic external defibrillators (AEDs): fully automatic and semiautomatic. A semi-automatic AED requires the EMT to hook up two defibrillatory patches to the patient's chest, connect the leads, and turn on the AED. The fully automatic AED will initiate shock automatically.

126. The answer is B. (Mosby, Cardiovascular Emergencies) Once the semiautomatic AED is hooked up to the patient and turned on, the user presses a button to have the unit analyze the cardiac rhythm. The computer then advises which steps to take, based on its analysis of the patient's cardiac rhythm. The user delivers the shocks manually by pressing a button, if so advised.

127. The answer is C. (Brady, Cardiac Emergencies) AEDs are designed to shock patients in both ventricular fibrillation and ventricular tachycardia. While every patient in ventricular fibrillation is in cardiac arrest, that is not the case for ventricular tachycardia. Some patients with ventricular tachycardia are in cardiac arrest (unconscious, pulseless, and apneic) and will benefit from defibrillation by an AED; some have a pulse and are conscious, and should not be defibrillated.

128. The answer is D. (Mosby Cardiovascular Emergencies) Before attaching a patient to an AED it is essential to make sure that the patient is in cardiac arrest (unconscious, pulseless, and apneic). If a patient is in ventricular tachycardia, the AED will detect it and advise shocking the patient, regardless of whether the patient has a pulse. Shocking a patient in ventricular tachycardia who has a pulse may cause the patient to go into ventricular fibrillation or asystole and thus put the patient in cardiac arrest.

129. The answer is D. (Mosby, Cardiovascular Emergencies) Before attaching the AED it is essential to make sure that the patient is in cardiac arrest (pulseless, apneic, and unconscious). It is appropriate to shock a patient in ventricular tachycardia who is in cardiac arrest. The other situations listed in the question may result in a patient being shocked inappropriately.

130. The answer is B. (Mosby, Cardiovascular Emergencies) If a patient is in water, the patient should be moved to a dry place and any wet clothing should be taken off before an AED is attached to the patient. Similarly, a patient who is touching a metal object should be moved out of contact with it before an AED is attached. These precautions prevent other people who are touching the water or metal from getting a shock when the AED is turned on.

131. The answer is A. (Mosby, Cardiovascular Emergencies) In the cardiac arrest patient defibrillation takes priority over CPR. Therefore, a lone EMT-Basic should use the AED to analyze the need for defibrillation before instituting CPR. CPR is stopped before turning on the AED, to ensure proper rhythm identification and to prevent the person performing CPR from getting shocked. CPR may be stopped for up to 90 seconds while three consecutive shocks are delivered.

132. The answer is D. (Mosby, Cardiovascular Emergencies) CPR should be stopped while the AED analyzes the heart rhythm and while shocks are being delivered. The movements of the patient that occur during CPR may cause the AED to misread the rhythm. Anyone touching the patient when the AED delivers a shock may also get shocked. CPR may be stopped for up to 90 seconds while three consecutive shocks are delivered.

133. The answer is D. (AAOS, Cardiac Emergencies) With a fully automatic AED, all the operator has to do is to connect the defibrillatory pads and cables to the patient and turn on the power. The device analyzes the heart rhythm and delivers a shock automatically.

134. The answer is B. (AAOS, Cardiac Emergencies) The semiautomatic AED has the advantages listed in choices A, C, and D. In addition, the device often has a manual control module that allows the operator to administer a shock for cardiac rhythms other than the ones for which the device is programmed to recommend defibrillation. The device is usually faster to operate (less than 1 minute) than a manual defibrillator.

135. The answer is B. (AAOS, Cardiac Emergencies) The fully automated defibrillator's sensitivity is a major problem. If the patient is touched or moved while the machine is analyzing the heart rhythm, the machine sees ventricular fibrillation and shocks the patient.

136. The answer is B. (Mosby, Cardiovascular Emergencies) A fully automatic AED can usually deliver its first shock within 1 minute of arrival at the patient's side. This is sometimes faster than a shock can be delivered by a paramedic with a manual defribrillator.

137. The answer is C. (Mosby, Cardiovascular Emergencies) Before using an AED and after taking appropriate body substance isolation precautions, it is essential first to confirm that the patient is in cardiac arrest—that is, apneic, unconscious, and pulseless. Once cardiac arrest is confirmed, CPR is begun (or resumed) while the operator starts applying the AED electrodes. Only then is the AED turned on.

138. The answer is A. (AAOS, Cardiac Emergencies) While the features listed in choices B, C, and D are all advantages of using an AED, they will only assist the operator in treating the cardiac rhythms for which the AED is programmed to recommend defibrillation—ventricular fibrillation and ventricular tachycardia (usually with a heart rate faster than 180 beats per minute). The manual control module allows the operator (physician or paramedic) to shock patients with other types of cardiac rhythm.

139. The answer is C. (Mosby, Cardiovascular Emergencies) Manual defibrillators, which can be used by paramedics, have "hands-on" defibrillator paddles. The "hand-off" adhesive defibrillation pads used with an AED are safer for the operator.

140. The answer is B. (Brady, Cardiac Emergencies) After attaching the AED, it is essential to stop CPR, because any patient movement may cause a false rhythm analysis. At the same time, all individuals must be clear from contact with the patient and with all equipment attached to the patient. In the event that a shock is advised and given, this precaution will prevent other individuals from being shocked as well.

141. The answer is C. (Brady, Cardiac Emergencies) In treating a cardiac arrest patient with an AED, when the patient remains continuously in a "shock indicated" rhythm, a total of six shocks are to be administered. If, after six shocks, a pulse is still absent, then you should resume CPR and transport the patient. If, however, a pulse is present you should monitor vital signs and transport.

142. The answer is D. (Mosby, Cardiovascular Emergencies) If a successfully shocked patient with a pulse again becomes pulseless, apneic, and unresponsive, then the EMT-Basic should proceed as in choice D. Advanced cardiac life support (ACLS) backup should also be called for.

143. The answer is B. (Mosby, Cardiovascular Emergencies) In administering AED-advised shocks in two sets of three stacked shocks, pulse checks are only performed after shock 3 and shock 6. Only AED rhythm analysis is performed between shocks 1 and 2, 2 and 3, 4 and 5, and 5 and 6.

144. The answer is D. (AAOS, Cardiac Emergencies) While choices A through C are standard reasons to begin transport, your local medical protocol may establish its own criteria for treatment and transport of the cardiac arrest patient. Local medical protocols may permit additional shocks and/or provide immediate advanced cardiac life support (ACLS) backup or even air transport.

145. **The answer is C.** (AAOS, Cardiac Emergencies) While choices A, B, and D all represent correct treatment options, choice D is the least preferred, because performing CPR in a moving ambulance is inadequate, difficult, and dangerous.

146. **The answer is A.** (Mosby, Cardiovascular Emergencies) Because, in every cardiac arrest patient, defibrillation should always be the first step, preceding CPR, choice A gives the correct sequence. However, in every cardiac arrest patient, before attaching and operating the AED, it is essential to take body substance isolation precautions and to confirm that the patient is unresponsive, pulseless, and apneic.

147. **The answer is C.** (AAOS, Cardiac Emergencies) Because a series of three "stacked" shocks result in a better chance of successful defibrillation, many AEDs are programmed to do this without you even needing to press the *Analyze* button between shocks. Other AEDs still require you to press a button to analyze the rhythm after each shock.

148. **The answer is D.** (AAOS, Cardiac Emergencies) The chain of survival has four links— early EMS access, early CPR, early defibrillation, and early ACLS. ALS units provide early ACLS, including intubation and intravenous medications. These ACLS maneuvers may improve the success rate of resuscitation.

149. **The answer is C.** (AAOS, Cardiac Emergencies) Postresuscitation care include choices A, B, and D. ALS backup will provide endotracheal intubation and intravenous medications, which may improve the success of resuscitation. After an EMT-Basic successfully defibrillates a patient, the patient, with a pulse, may receive intravenous medications to prevent a recurrence of cardiac arrest. All postresuscitation patients must be transported with high concentration of oxygen.

150. **The answer is C.** (AAOS, Cardiac Emergencies) At present, an EMT-Basic is required to maintain AED skills by refresher training every 3 months. However, state laws and local medical direction may set additional requirements or guidelines for maintaining this skill.

151. **The answer is C.** (Mosby, Cardiovascular Emergencies) At present, EMT-Basics must complete an "Operator's Shift Checklist for Automated Defibrillators" on a daily basis. The American Heart Association publishes additional guidelines on AEDs.

152. **The answer is D.** (Mosby, Cardiovascular Emergencies) The American Heart Association, through its basic life support (BLS-CPR) and advanced cardiac life support (ACLS) courses, has educated the medical community and public concerning the importance of early defibrillation. This education has also been accomplished through the efforts listed in choices A through C, among others.

153. **The answer is D.** (AAOS, Cardiac Emergencies) In addition to the reasons given in choices A through C, case review also provides an opportunity to go over additional aspects of the care provided to the patient. This would include the proper use of oxygen, airway adjuncts, the written report, and postresuscitation care. Finally, it is emotionally draining to participate in the resuscitation of another human being. You should benefit from being able to openly discuss all aspects of the care given to your patient.

154. **The answer is B.** (AAOS, Cardiac Emergencies) The role of the medical director includes the activities listed in choices A, C, and D, as well as the evaluation of the quality of basic life support and advanced life support provided by the system for all types of emergencies (not just cardiac arrest).

155. **The answer is A.** (Mosby, Cardiovascular Emergencies) The primary goal of quality improvement in an EMS system in which EMT-Basics use AEDs is to provide the best quality of patient care. By carefully reviewing all aspects of the care in each case, individual and system changes may be instituted to improve the survival outcomes of cardiac arrest patients.

156. **The answer is A.** (AAOS, Cardiac Emergencies) The most common reason for the failure of an AED's event recorder is battery failure. The battery should be replaced at least once a day.

157. **The answer is C.** (AAOS, Cardiac Emergencies) The roles of medical direction in the provision of emergency medical care for the chest-pain patient include those listed in choices A, B, and D, as well as constant quality improvement of the entire EMS system.

158. **The answer is B.** (Brady, Diabetic Emergencies/Alt Mental Status) Hypoglycemia (low blood sugar) may cause many different conditions in a patient, including those listed in choices A, C, and D. It may also cause a patient to appear intoxicated, have slurred speech, cold clammy skin, rapid heart rate, hunger, seizures, anxiety, and other uncharacteristic behavior. However, it should not cause low blood pressure.

159. **The answer is B.** (Brady, Diabetic Emergencies/Alt Mental Status) Some of the most helpful ways of establishing that a patient with an altered mental status has diabetes are those listed in choices A, C, and D. Patients with an altered mental status from any cause (drugs, alcohol, stroke, etc.) may react angrily to questions concerning medical history.

160. **The answer is A.** (Mosby, Diabetic/Alt Mental Status) In assessing a patient on diabetic medication with an altered mental status, it is important to check for any clues as to why a hypoglycemic (low blood sugar) reaction may be occurring. The reason may include skipping a meal, vomiting a meal, extra-vigorous exercise (which burns off glucose), and accidentally

or purposely taking too much diabetic medication. Physical examination may reveal other signs consistent with a hypoglycemic reaction—cold, clammy skin or a rapid heartbeat.

161. The answer is D. (Mosby, Diabetic/Alt Mental Status) In patients with altered mental status, airway management is of prime concern because of the reasons listed in choices A through C. Inability to manage the airway correctly may lead to additional medical complications, such as obstructed airway, aspiration of secretions or vomit into the lungs producing pneumonia, or hypoxia (low blood oxygen), which may worsen the mental status or lead to heart arrhythmias. Patients with altered mental status do not frequently have anatomically abnormal airways.

162. The answer is B. (Mosby, Diabetic/Alt Mental Status) These are two of the trade names for oral glucose preparations, which EMT-Basics may administer to diabetic patients with altered mental status, with medical direction approval. The preparations in choice A, along with humulin regular and NPH insulin, are injections administered to lower the blood glucose (sugar) level in the blood in diabetic patients. The preparations listed in choices C and D, along with Glucotrol, Glynase, and Tolinase, are examples of oral hypoglycemic agents, which are prescribed for diabetic patients to lower their blood glucose levels.

163. The answer is D. (Mosby, Diabetic/Alt Mental Status) The guidelines in choices A through C are essential parts of the EMT-Basics administration of oral glucose to a confirmed diabetic patient with an altered mental status. After administering oral glucose, it is essential to perform ongoing assessments every 5 minutes.

164. The answer is D. (AAOS, Diabetic Emergencies) In administering oral glucose to a diabetic patient with an altered mental status, the statements in choices A through C are true. However, administering oral glucose to alert patients is not dangerous.

165. The answer is A. (Mosby, Allergic Reactions) A patient suffering an allergic reaction may complain of all of the symptoms in choices B, C, and D, as well as difficulty breathing, hoarseness, palpitations, watery eyes, headache, a feeling of impending doom, and confusion. While low blood pressure may result from an allergic reaction it is a sign rather than a symptom—that is, it is a manifestation that can be observed by someone other than the patient, rather than a sensation that can be felt and reported only by the patient.

166. The answer is D. (AAOS, Allergies and Poisoning) Signs of an allergic reaction include those listed in choices A through C, as well as watery eyes; runny nose; hives; stridor; horseness; flushed skin; rash; rapid pulse; swelling of the face, tongue, neck, hands and feet; and cardiac arrest. Headache can be a symptom of an allergic reaction, but it is not a sign.

167. The answer is B. (Mosby, Allergic Reactions) While B represents the mechanism, other signs of respiratory distress may be seen in allergic reactions, such as wheezing, tight chest with distant breath sounds, and respiratory arrest. A and C are signs of an allergic reaction but are not part of the mechanism of progressive respiratory distress. D is a cause of respiratory distress but is unrelated to an allergic reaction.

168. The answer is A. (Mosby, Allergic Reactions) B and C are clearly part of an EMT-Basic's emergency care of a patient with a severe allergic reaction. D would only apply to patients in whom assessment revealed respiratory distress or hypoperfusion (low blood pressure). A is frequently part of the treatment plan for severe allergic reactions by emergency department physicians and sometimes paramedics, but it is not part of the emergency care given by an EMT-Basic.

169. The answer is D. (Mosby, Allergic Reactions) There is no contraindication to the use of an epinephrine injection in a patient suffering a life-threatening allergic reaction, identification of which includes demonstrating respiratory distress or hypoperfusion (low blood pressure). However, since epinephrine may significantly elevate the patient's blood pressure and pulse rate, you should continuously monitor your patient while administering oxygen and instituting rapid transport.

170. The answer is C. (AAOS, Allergies and Poisoning) C describes the correct sequence to follow. It is also important to record that you gave the injection and the time. Finally, you need to dispose of the auto-injector in the proper biohazard container. Choices A and B are incorrect because they give the wrong location on the thigh. Choice D is incorrect because the injector should be held in place until the medication is injected.

171. The answer is A. (Mosby, Poisoning/Overdose) Along with oral ingestion of poisons, which include drugs, alcohol, household products, contaminated foods, and plants, B, C, and D are the other ways that poisons may enter the body. A is incorrect because liquid toxins cannot evaporate through a closed bottle and reach the body to cause poisoning.

172. The answer is B. (Mosby, Poisoning/Overdose) While A, C, and D correctly identify possible signs and symptoms of the accompanying type of poisoning, B does not. Injected toxins may produce weakness, dizziness, chills, fever, nausea, and vomiting.

173. The answer is C. (Mosby, Poisoning Overdose) The emergency medical care of a suspected ingested overdose may include the actions listed in choices A, B, and D. While contacting medical control to request the physician's order to administer activated charcoal to a suspected ingested overdose is usually correct, unconsciousness (altered mental status) is one of the contraindications to administering it. The other contraindications are suspected acid or alkali ingestion, inability to swallow, and active seizures.

174. The answer is D. (Mosby, Poisoning/Overdose) While A, B, and C are correct, D is not. The side effects of activated charcoal are black stools and vomiting.

175. The answer is D. (Mosby, Poisoning/Overdose) A, B, and C are all trade names for activated charcoal. D is not.

176. **The answer is C.** (Mosby, Poisoning/Overdose) The emergency medical care of the patient suffering from injected toxins may include the measures in choices A, B, and D. However, the EMT-Basic should not attempt to catch a venomous snake or spider for identification or testing. If the spider is dead, however, you should bring it to the hospital.

177. **The answer is A.** (Mosby, Poisoning/Overdose) While B, C, and D are all correct, A is not. It is essential to obtain an order from medical direction to administer activated charcoal before giving it.

178. **The answer is B.** (Brady, Environmental Emergencies) A, C, and D are correct definitions of ways in which the body loses heat; respiration is another way, involving the loss of body heat with exhaled warm air. While convection is a way for the body to lose heat, the definition in choice B is incorrect. Heat lost by convection is heat lost to currents of air or water that pass over the body.

179. **The answer is C.** (Brady, Environmental Emergencies) A, B, and D are some of the signs of hypothermia. C is incorrect because the abdominal skin temperature is cool in the hypothermic patient.

180. **The answer is C.** (Brady, Environmental Emergencies) A, B, and D are correct examples of changing sings and symptoms of hypothermia. C is incorrect because, in the early stages of hypothermia, a patient usually has rapid breathing and a rapid pulse. In later stages of hypothermia, the patient has slow to absent breathing, slow to absent pulse, and low to absent blood pressure.

181. **The answer is B.** (Mosby, Environmental Emergencies) A, C, and D, as well as not allowing the patient to walk or become active, are part of the emergency care for an alert hypothermic patient. B is incorrect; you should always remove wet clothing and then cover the patient in warm blankets.

182. **The answer is C.** (Mosby, Environmental Emergencies) A, B, D, and not allowing the patient to walk or become active are part of the emergency care for the hypothermic patient with a decreased level of responsiveness. C is incorrect, because actively rewarming a severely hypothermic patient may cause life-threatening heart arrhythmias.

183. **The answer is D.** (Mosby, Environmental Emergencies) A, B, and C, as well as covering the patient with warm blankets and turning up the heat in the patient compartment of the ambulance, are all part of the emergency care for the hypothermic patient with no signs of life. D is incorrect because, in a hypothermic patient with no sings of life, you should check for a pulse for 30 to 45 seconds before starting CPR.

184. **The answer is A.** (Mosby, Environmental Emergencies) B, C, and D, as well as weakness or exhaustion, dizziness or fainting, a rapid or pounding heartbeat, nausea and vomiting, and abdominal cramps, are all signs and symptoms of hyperthermia. Frequent urination is not related to hyperthermia.

185. **The answer is C.** (Brady, Environmental Emergencies) A, B, and D are part of the emergency care rendered to a hyperthermic patient with moist, pale, normal-to-cool skin. In addition, administering oxygen, allowing a responsive patient to drink water, keeping an unresponsive or vomiting patient lying on the left side, and applying moist towels over cramped muscles are also part of the emergency care. C is incorrect; the patient should be kept at rest in the supine position with legs elevated.

186. **The answer is A.** (Brady, Environmental Emergencies) B, C, and D are all part of the emergency care of the hyperthermic patient with skin that is hot and either dry or moist. Also, if transport is delayed, the patient should be immersed up to the neck in a tub or container of cool water, while the vitals signs are monitored. A is incorrect, because all hyperthermic patients should be given oxygen by a non-rebreather mask.

187. **The answer is A.** (Brady, Environmental Emergencies) A patient suffering from heat exposure whose skin is hot and either dry or moist represents a true emergency. This condition is often referred to as *heat stroke*. If the skin is moist and pale and either cool or normal in temperature, the condition is less serious. The condition is known as *heat exhaustion*.

188. **The answer is C.** (Brady, Environmental Emergencies) A, B, and D, as well as cardiac arrest, signs of a heart attack, internal injuries, and drowning or near-drowning, are all common in water-related emergencies. Hyperthermia is not; prolonged exposure to cold water will cause hypothermia, however.

189. **The answer is D.** (Mosby, Environmental Emergencies) A, B, and C, as well as cardiac arrest, are complications of near-drowning. The incidence of spinal injuries in this situation is very high. Therefore, any unresponsive patient in the water should be immobilized on a long board while the head is stabilized manually. Skin rash is unrelated to near-drowning as such.

190. **The answer is C.** (Mosby, Environmental Emergencies) A, B, and D, as well as proper removal of any stinger and washing of the area, are all part of emergency medical care for bites and stings. In the case of snake bites, medical control should be consulted concerning the use of constricting bands. C is incorrect because, if the injury is to an extremity, it should be positioned below the level of the heart.

191. **The answer is B.** (Mosby, Environmental Emergencies) B is the correct way to remove a stinger from the skin. A, C, and D are all incorrect because they all can squeeze venom out of a venom sac still attached to the stinger.

192. **The answer is A.** (Brady, Behavioral Emergencies) A is the most complete definition of a behavioral emergency. A patient who represents a true behavioral emergency may satisfy only a portion of this definition. The types of behavior described in the other choices do not in themselves represent behavioral emergencies.

193. **The answer is D.** (Brady, Behavioral Emergencies) A, B, and C are good examples of general factors and medical conditions that may result in alteration of a patient's behavior. There are may others, such as sepsis (generalized infection), meningitis (infection in the brain or spinal cord), and an overactive or underactive thryoid gland. Skin rash and hair loss should not result in any alteration of a patient's behavior by themselves.

194. **The answer is D.** (Mosby, Behavioral Emergencies) A, B, and C are some of the most common psychiatric disorders that may cause a patient to have a psychological crisis. While insomnia may be a significant stress on any patient, it usually does not cause a psychological crisis.

195. **The answer is A.** (Brady, Behavioral Emergencies) B, C, and D, as well as depression, high stress levels, alcohol and drug abuse, and certain ages (high suicide rates occur at the ages of 15 to 25 and over the age of 40) are all characteristics suggestive of a suicidal patient. A family history of suicide for adopted parents does not increase an individual's risk of suicide.

196. **The answer is C.** (Brady, Behavioral Emergencies) A, B, and D are all reasonable components of providing treatment and transport of a patient with a behavioral emergency. Restraining patients against their will is usually initiated by law enforcement authorities. However, gagging a patient's mouth is never an acceptable part of the restraining procedure.

197. **The answer is B.** (Mosby, Behavioral Emergencies) In responding to every call for emergency medical care, particularly behavioral emergencies, it is essential to perform a "scene size-up." This is done to make sure that the scene is safe for you and your partner. If it is unsafe, do not enter. In this case, the patient appears hostile and has an unsafe object—a knife—next to him. Therefore, answer B is correct. A, C, and D are incorrect since the scene is unsafe. A is also incorrect since law enforcement officers should handle disarming a patient. C is also incorrect because you try not to allow the patient between you and the nearest exit. D is also incorrect since you never want to provoke or agitate a hostile patient.

198. **The answer is D.** (Mosby, Behavioral Emergencies) A, B, and C, as well as sitting on the edge of a seat, throwing objects, yelling and using foul language, and any behavior that makes the EMT uneasy, are all signs of possible violent behavior on the part of the patient. D is not.

199. **The answer is C.** (Brady, Behavioral Emergencies) A, B, and D are all methods that are helpful in trying to calm the patient. No matter how verbally abusive or angry the patient becomes, it is essential to remain calm. C is incorrect, because most patients with behavioral emergencies need to be approached in a calm, unhurried manner and encouraged slowly to accept assistance.

200. The answer is A. (AAOS, Obstetrics and Gynecology) Retained placenta is a complication that may occur *after* the delivery of an infant; it is not a predelivery condition. B, C, and D, as well as trauma to a pregnant woman and unborn fetus, are all predelivery emergencies.

201. (Mosby, Obstetrics and Gynecology)

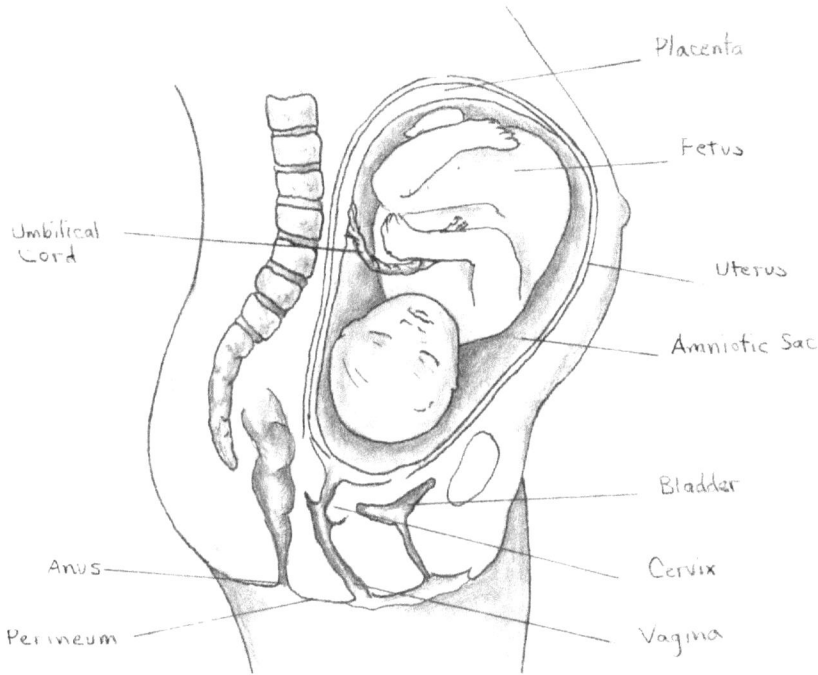

Placenta
Fetus
Umbilical Cord
Uterus
Amniotic Sac
Bladder
Anus
Cervix
Perineum
Vagina

202. The answer is D. (Mosby, Obstetrics and Gynecology) A, B, C are all contents of the obstetrics kit with correct descriptions of their use. Other contents and their use are:

> A bulb syringe, used to suction the infant's nose & mouth
> Towels, used to dry the infant
> 2 × 10 gauze sponges, used to wipe the infants mouth and nose
> One baby blanket, used to warm the infant
> Sanitary napkins, for the mother after delivery
> A plastic bag ,used to transport the placenta to the hospital

D is incorrect because the sterile gloves in the kit are to be worn throughout delivery and for the care of the newborn infant.

203. The answer is C. (AAOS, Obstetrics and Gynecology) A, B, and D are parts of emergency care given to a patient having a miscarriage. If the patient demonstrates any signs of shock, she should be transported lying on her left side. C is incorrect, because you *never* try to pull any tissue out of the vagina.

204. The answer is C. (Mosby, Obstetrics and Gynecology) A, B, and D are all indications that the delivery is imminent. The mother may also say that she feels increasing pressure in the vaginal area and in the rectum, which feels like a bowel movement. Tingling in the lower legs may occur but is not a sign of an imminent delivery.

205. **The answer is C.** (AAOS, Obstetrics and Gynecology) Body substance isolation precautions are essential in dealing with any patient with vaginal bleeding. A is incorrect, because the patient is not in labor and is not having an imminent delivery. B is incorrect, because, with a blood pressure of 74/50, she is showing a sign of shock and needs to lie on her left side, which will help with the return of blood from her legs to her heart. D is incorrect, since you need to save all bloodied sanitary pads, so that the hospital staff can estimate the amount of blood loss.

206. **The answer is B.** (Brady, Obstetrics and Gynecology) A, C, and D, as well as keeping the patient warm (but not overheated), and having an obstetrics kit ready, are all a part of the emergency care of a pregnant seizing patient. B is incorrect, because a seizing or postictal (post-seizing) patient is usually unconscious and unable to protect her airway. Should the patient vomit, she would aspirate the vomit into her lungs. You must be prepared to suction the seizing or postictal patient who begins to vomit.

207. **The answer is C.** (Brady, Obstetrics and Gynecology) As a trauma victim with a possible spinal injury, this patient must have her spine immobilized as the first priority. The board and patient are then tipped to the left to take pressure off of the abdominal organs and vena cava. A, B, and D are routine parts of the emergency care of a pregnant female with any predelivery emergency and thus are not unique to the situation described here (trauma with a possible spinal injury).

208. **The answer is C.** (Brady, Obstetrics and Gynecology) A, B, and D, as well as trying to provide privacy for the mother and positioning the obstetrics kit on a nearby table or chair, are all important steps in predelivery preparation. C is incorrect because, at the mother's choice, the father, the mother's assistant, or one member of the delivery team should always be placed by the mother's head. This person's role is to provide emotional support and to be prepared to turn the mother's head to the side should she vomit.

209. **The answer is C.** (Brady, Obstetrics and Gynecology) A, B, and D are all part of the steps in assisting the mother with the delivery of her infant. In addition, after the baby's head delivers, you should check the baby's airway and suction the baby's mouth, then the nose. Then you help deliver the baby's shoulders. After the feet are delivered, you again suction the baby's mouth, then nose. Finally, you wrap the infant in a warm, dry blanket and record the exact time of birth. C is incorrect because, if the amniotic sac has not broken, you would use your finger to puncture the membrane.

210. **The answer is A.** (Brady, Obstetrics and Gynecology) B, C, and D, as well as one under the vagina, are the correct positions for sheets or towels in preparing the mother for an imminent delivery.

211. The answer is C. (Brady, Obstetrics and Gynecology) C is the only correct initial approach to the problem of delivering an infant with the umbilical cord wrapped around the baby's neck. A and B are both incorrect and dangerous to the infant. D is incorrect because it is not the initial approach to the treatment of this problem. However, if you are unsuccessful in attempting to perform C, you should not attempt to deliver the baby, until after D is performed.

212. The answer is A. (Mosby, Obstetrics and Gynecology) A is the correct treatment of the newly delivered baby's head. B is incorrect, because you should put gentle pressure against the baby's head during crowning to prevent an extremely rapid or explosive birth. This will help prevent tearing of the mother's perineum. You never put traction on the baby's head during delivery. C is incorrect because you need to support the delivered baby's head for the remainder of the delivery. You also need to wipe and suction the mouth and nose right away. D is incorrect because you support the baby's delivered head as it naturally rotates and then immediately wipe and suction the baby's mouth and nose.

213. The answer is D. (Brady, Obstetrics and Gynecology) D represents the correct time to clamp and cut the umbilical cord. A and B are incorrect because there is no exact time (in minutes) to clamp and cut the cord; the time is decided by the two clinical criteria given in D. C is incorrect because the baby should never be bathed in the prehospital setting, only after arrival at the medical facility. Also, the delivery of the placenta has nothing to do with the clamping and cutting of the cord. (Usually the placenta is delivered within a few minutes after the clamping and cutting of the umbilical cord.)

214. The answer is C. (Brady, Obstetrics and Gynecology) A, B, and D all represent correct steps in the cutting of the umbilical cord. It is essential to not cut a pulsating umbilical cord. It is also important to not cut the umbilical cord of a baby who is not breathing, unless you need to remove the cord from around the neck or you have to perform CPR. C is incorrect because you should cut the umbilical cord between the two clamps, to minimize the bleeding. If the cord is not completely closed, the baby could possibly bleed to death.

215. The answer is A. (Brady, Obstetrics and Gynecology) B, C, and D are all true statements concerning the delivery of the placenta. The afterbirth is made up of the placenta, the umbilical cord, the membranes of the amniotic sac, and some tissues lining the uterus. A is incorrect because, in most cases, the placenta is expelled within a few minutes after the baby is born.

216. The answer is C. (AAOS, Obstetrics and Gynecology) A newborn infant usually begins breathing on its own within a few seconds of birth.

217. The answer is B. (AAOS, Obstetrics and Gynecology) A, C, and D are all part of post-delivery emergency medical care. B is incorrect, since you should never digitally examine the vagina or put anything in it, because doing so may cause additional injury or introduce infection.

218. **The answer is C.** (Brady, Obstetrics and Gynecology) A, B, and D represent the correct sequence of caring for a newborn baby who does not begin breathing on its own. There is no indication for slapping a baby's buttocks to stimulate breathing.

219. **The answer is D.** (Mosby, Obstetrics and Gynecology) A, B, and C are all correct components of neonatal resuscitation. D is incorrect because free-flow oxygen is administered by holding an oxygen mask or tubing as close as possible to the newborn's mouth and nose, not inside the mouth.

220. **The answer is A.** (Mosby, Obstetrics and Gynecology) Evaluating the heart rate is the next step to take in resuscitating a newborn after you have begun artificial ventilations. It is essential at that point to determine whether the infant requires external cardiac chest compression. Suctioning of the airway and stimulation with back rubbing and heel flicks were already tried and do not need to be repeated. Calling medical control may be helpful, but the first priority is to evaluate the nonbreathing infant's heart rate.

221. **The answer is B.** (Brady, Obstetrics and Gynecology) A, C, and D are all parts of the emergency care for assisting a mother with a breech delivery. A breech delivery is one in which the head is delivered last. The baby's legs or buttocks deliver first. In addition, if, during the breech delivery, the body delivers, you must provide support to it and prevent an explosive delivery of the head. B is incorrect because, in a legs-first breech delivery, you never should pull on the baby's legs.

222. **The answer is D.** (Mosby, Obstetrics and Gynecology) A, B, and C are correct actions in caring for a breech delivery with an undelivered head. If the head still does not deliver, you should transport immediately while maintaining the V-position. D is incorrect because, in a breech delivery, you should never pull on the legs, buttocks, or trunk.

223. **The answer is C.** (Brady, Obstetrics and Gynecology) A prolapsed cord is an emergency because the cord may be squeezed shut between the baby's head and the vaginal wall, cutting off the baby's supply of blood and thus of oxygen. A and B are incorrect because prolapse of the umbilical cord does not lead to infection or recurrent vomiting by the baby. D is incorrect because you never reinsert a prolapsed umbilical cord into the vagina.

224. **The answer is B.** (AAOS, Obstetrics and Gynecology) The best signs that there is an additional baby (or babies) to be delivered is that the mother's abdomen remains large after the delivery, and/or the first baby is small, and/or the mother begins to feel strong contractions about 10 minutes after the first birth. Another reliable sign is if the mother tells you that a sonogram showed she was carrying twins. The second baby may deliver before or after the delivery of the first baby's placenta.

225. **The answer is A.** (AAOS, Obstetrics and Gynecology) The color of meconium-stained amniotic fluid is usually green or brownish yellow. The other choices are all true statements.

226. **The answer is C.** (Mosby, Obstetrics and Gynecology) A, B, and D are all part of the emergency medical care of the premature infant. It is also important to transport the infant to a hospital equipped to provide neonatal resuscitation. C is incorrect because the bleeding umbilical cord should be clamped a second time, closer to the infant. The first clamp should not be removed.

227. **The answer is A.** (AAOS, Obstetrics and Gynecology) B, C, and D, as well as ensuring and maintaining the patient's airway, treating the patient for shock, and providing rapid transport, are all part of the emergency care of a patient in shock due to vaginal bleeding. A is incorrect because you never should pack or place dressings in the vagina.

228. **The answer is D.** (AAOS, Obstetrics and Gynecology) Soothing the patient during transport is often the key part of the treatment of a sexual assault victim. You should not examine the genitalia unless bleeding requires the application of a dressing. You should also encourage the patient not to wash, douche, urinate, or defecate until after a physician examines the patient. This is essential in order to best preserve evidence of the assault. C is not correct because the patient has the right to refuse assistance and transport to the emergency department.

TRAUMA

Directions: Each item below contains four suggested responses. Select the **one best** response to each item.

229. If bleeding from an upper extremity is not controlled by direct pressure, you should next

   (A) apply a tourniquet
   (B) elevate the extremity
   (C) apply the pneumatic antishock garment and inflate all compartments
   (D) remove the dressing and inspect the wound

230. A trauma patient has a blood pressure of 110/60, a pulse of 108, and a respiratory rate of 24. The patient complains of severe thirst and asks for some water to drink. You should

   (A) give the patient small sips of water
   (B) give the patient as much water as desired
   (C) give the patient small sips of brandy or another alcoholic beverage
   (D) allow the patient to suck on a piece of moistened gauze

231. You must carefully monitor the pressure in the pneumatic antishock garment for a patient who is

   (A) very obese
   (B) less than 66 inches tall
   (C) secured to a long spine board
   (D) being transported by helicopter

232. A true statement concerning internal bleeding is that it

   (A) is usually not serious
   (B) can be easily controlled in the field
   (C) is most often fatal
   (D) usually requires surgery or intensive hospital care

233. Shock causes damage to the body by means of

(A) inadequate blood flow to the organs
(B) ruptured blood vessels
(C) hypertension
(D) an excess number of red blood cells

234. The pneumatic antishock garment, once applied and inflated,

(A) should be removed if the patient's condition deteriorates
(B) should be removed if the patient's condition improves
(C) should be removed if the patient complains of pain
(D) should not be removed in the field

235. Bruising on the abdomen is a sign of

(A) internal bleeding
(B) shock
(C) minor injury
(D) melena

236. A systolic blood pressure of less than 90 mm Hg in an adult trauma patient is a sign of

(A) compensated shock
(B) decompensated shock
(C) hypertension
(D) head injury

237. A tourniquet should be applied in which of the following locations?

(A) Over an arterial pressure point
(B) As far proximal as possible on the limb
(C) Proximal to the wound, but as far distal as possible on the limb
(D) Distal to the wound

238. An effective way to control nosebleed is to

(A) pack the nose with dry sterile gauze
(B) pack the nose with moist sterile gauze
(C) have the patient sit quietly with the head tilted back as far as possible
(D) apply direct pressure by pinching the fleshy part of the patient's nostrils together

239. Bright red blood that spurts from a wound in time with the patient's pulse is a sign of

(A) bleeding from an artery
(B) bleeding from a vein
(C) bleeding from a capillary
(D) internal bleeding

240. Bleeding from most wounds will typically

(A) stop immediately on its own
(B) stop within 1 minute on its own
(C) stop in 6 to 20 minutes on its own
(D) not stop without treatment

241. You have responded to a patient who has fallen approximately 30 feet from a scaffold. The patient responds only to pain and has rapid snoring respirations. He appears pale, and his skin is cool and moist. His blood pressure is 80/50, and respiratory rate is 24. Your first treatment is to

(A) establish and maintain an airway with a jaw thrust
(B) establish and maintain an airway with the head-tilt/chin-lift
(C) apply a pneumatic antishock garment and inflate all compartments
(D) administer high-concentration oxygen

242. Almost all instances of external bleeding can be controlled most effectively by

(A) applying the pneumatic antishock garment
(B) applying a tourniquet
(C) applying pressure to an arterial pressure point
(D) applying direct pressure to the wound

243. Once you have controlled bleeding with direct pressure, you should

(A) remove the dressing and inspect the wound
(B) apply a tourniquet proximal to the wound
(C) maintain pressure on the wound by securing the dressing with a roller bandage
(D) apply pressure to an arterial pressure point

244. Elevation of an extremity with a bleeding wound

(A) may help to slow or stop the bleeding
(B) will usually increase the bleeding
(C) will make it very difficult to apply direct pressure to the wound
(D) should only be attempted when all other methods have failed

245. Which of the following should never be used as a tourniquet?

(A) A triangular bandage
(B) A length of rope
(C) A blood pressure cuff
(D) A bandage that is 4 inches wide

246. All of the following are major functions of the skin EXCEPT

(A) protection from infection
(B) temperature regulation
(C) maintenance of water balance
(D) production of red blood cells

247. The layer of the skin that contains the nerve endings and special structures such as sweat glands is the

(A) epidermis
(B) dermis
(C) subcutaneous layer
(D) fascia

248. The first step in treating all open wounds is to

(A) control bleeding by direct pressure
(B) apply a pressure bandage
(C) clean the wound surface of major contamination
(D) employ appropriate body sub-stance isolation techniques

249. A collection of blood that can be felt under the skin at the site of a closed wound is known as a

(A) contusion
(B) hematoma
(C) bruise
(D) hernia

250. If a patient has a bruise on the abdomen, the EMT-Basic should look for early signs of internal bleeding by

(A) palpating the abdomen
(B) measuring the blood pressure
(C) listening for breath sounds
(D) inducing the patient to vomit

251. All patients with suspected internal injuries should

(A) be transported lying in the left lateral recumbent position
(B) be given small sips of water
(C) be carefully monitored for signs of shock
(D) have a pneumatic antishock garment applied and inflated

252. A wound where a flap of skin is torn loose and only remains attached on one side is known as

(A) an abrasion
(B) a laceration
(C) a puncture
(D) an avulsion

253. Open wounds to the chest should be treated with

(A) a bulky gauze dressing
(B) no dressing
(C) an airtight dressing
(D) a loosely applied gauze dressing

254. If a patient appears to develop increasing respiratory distress, shock, and distended neck veins after being treated for an open chest wound you should

(A) decrease the amount of oxygen being administered
(B) position the patient to lie on the uninjured side
(C) raise the patient's head
(D) lift one corner of the airtight dressing

255. Patients with abdominal injuries should normally be transported

(A) in the prone position
(B) in the left lateral recumbent position
(C) with the head elevated
(D) in the supine position with the knees flexed

256. Organs protruding from the abdominal wall should be

(A) covered with a bulky dry dressing
(B) covered with a sterile dressing soaked with saline solution
(C) covered with a clean sheet
(D) left open to the air

257. A burn characterized by pain, reddening, and blisters is known as a

(A) superficial burn
(B) partial-thickness burn
(C) full-thickness burn
(D) third-degree burn

258. What is the percentage of the body surface area that is burned in an adult patient who has burns covering the entire left arm and the anterior and posterior chest?

(A) 18 percent
(B) 22.5 percent
(C) 27 percent
(D) 40 percent

259. Which of the following would be considered a critical burn?

(A) A partial-thickness burn of both feet
(B) A partial-thickness burn of the anterior right and left legs
(C) A partial-thickness burn of the anterior chest
(D) A full-thickness burn of the anterior upper arm

260. Extensive burns should be covered with

(A) dry sterile dressings
(B) wet sterile dressings
(C) commercial burn ointments
(D) airtight dressings

261. A burn caused by a caustic liquid should be

(A) immediately covered with a dry sterile dressing
(B) flushed briefly with water
(C) flushed with water for at least 20 minutes
(D) not treated until arrival at the hospital

262. The leakage of fluid and blood from damaged blood vessels after a blunt-force injury will cause a patient to experience

(A) numbness
(B) swelling and pain
(C) paralysis
(D) a burning sensation

263. If a patient has an extremity that is painful and swollen, you should suspect

(A) a sprain
(B) a dislocation
(C) a fracture
(D) any of the above

264. The purpose of splinting a painful, swollen, or deformed lower extremity is to

(A) set fractured bones
(B) allow free movement of broken bone ends
(C) allow the patient to walk
(D) immobilize the extremity to prevent further injury

265. Bleeding and swelling that results from a closed soft tissue injury to an extremity can best be controlled by

(A) application of cold, compression bandaging, elevation and splinting
(B) application of cold, splinting, and application of a tourniquet
(C) application of a pneumatic antishock garment
(D) application of heat and loose bandages

266. A serious complication that may result from an open painful, swollen, deformed extremity is

(A) paralysis
(B) infection
(C) hypothermia
(D) numbness

267. The sound or sensation that may be perceived when broken bone ends rub together is known as

(A) crepitus
(B) grinding
(C) deformity
(D) periostium

268. Signs of musculoskeletal injury include

(A) deformity
(B) loss of use
(C) discoloration
(D) all of the above

269. The first step in treating a patient with a painful, swollen, or deformed extremity is to

(A) assess pulses in the extremity
(B) apply a splint to the extremity
(C) apply a cold compress to the injury
(D) observe the appropriate body substance isolation precautions

270. The appropriate technique for an unstable multiple trauma patient with musculoskeletal injuries is to

(A) splint each affected extremity individually
(B) not splint the patient at all
(C) splint the patient's entire body with a spine board
(D) use a traction splint

271. A patient has a painful and severely deformed left lower leg. You should

(A) splint the leg in the position that you found it
(B) gently realign the limb prior to splinting it
(C) not apply a splint
(D) use a pillow splint

272. For a splint to be effective, it must immobilize

(A) only the affected bone
(B) the affected bone plus the joint above and the joint below it
(C) the affected bone and the joint above it
(D) the affected bone and the joint below it

273. The motion, sensation, and circulation of a painful, swollen, or deformed extremity should be assessed

(A) only before splinting the extremity
(B) only after splinting the extremity
(C) before and after splinting the extremity
(D) only if the patient complains of numbness

274. The most effective splint for use on injuries to the lower leg is the

(A) pillow splint
(B) rigid board splint
(C) traction splint
(D) sling and swathe

275. A pedestrian has been struck by an auto. As you approach the patient, you note a severe deformity to the left lower leg. Your first priority is to

(A) straighten the angulated leg to preserve circulation
(B) assess the circulation, sensation, and motor function distal to the leg injury
(C) splint the injured leg
(D) stabilize the patient's airway, breathing, and circulation

276. The EMT-Basic should apply manual traction to an injured extremity in order to

(A) reduce a fracture
(B) pull protruding bone ends back under the skin
(C) align the limb so that it can be splinted
(D) assess the circulation of a limb

277. When applying manual traction, the EMT-Basic should

(A) pull sharply along the long axis of the limb
(B) pull gently along the long axis of the limb
(C) push the limb sharply to one side
(D) push the limb gently to one side

278. When an EMT-Basic applies a traction splint, traction should be applied until

(A) the injured limb is longer than the other limb
(B) the patient feels discomfort
(C) the limb is maintained in the normal anatomic position
(D) the ratchet mechanism can no longer be tightened

279. A traction splint is most useful for

(A) a fractured forearm
(B) a dislocated shoulder
(C) a dislocated hip
(D) a fractured femur

280. Injuries to the elbow are considered serious because

(A) injuries at joints are difficult to splint properly
(B) the patient may experience more pain than with other injuries
(C) there may be life-threatening bleeding into the joint
(D) there is often damage to nearby nerves and blood vessels

281. Injuries to the hand should be splinted in the position of function by

(A) placing the hand flat on a rigid board
(B) forming the hand around a role of gauze or bulky dressing with the fingers slightly flexed
(C) having the patient make a tight fist prior to splinting
(D) using a traction splint

282. The primary danger of injuries to the pelvis is

(A) damage to the urinary bladder
(B) disability
(C) severe internal bleeding
(D) paralysis

283. A patient was involved in a side-impact motor vehicle accident. Assessment reveals pain and deformity to the left side of the pelvis. The patient appears pale, and vital signs are as follows: blood pressure 84/40, pulse 124, and respiratory rate 20. The most appropriate method of immobilization for this patient is a

(A) rigid splint
(B) long spine board
(C) pneumatic antishock garment
(D) traction splint

284. You have responded to a patient who fell from a ladder. The patient is complaining of pain in the right knee. Physical examination reveals a severe deformity at the right knee. You are unable to palpate a distal pulse in the foot, and the patient has no capillary refill in the toes. You should

(A) splint the knee in the position you found it in
(B) transport the patient without a splint
(C) make one attempt to realign the knee
(D) apply a traction splint

285. A pillow splint is most useful for injuries to the

(A) lower leg
(B) hand
(C) upper arm
(D) foot

286. An unconscious trauma patient should always be treated for

(A) internal bleeding
(B) spinal injury
(C) pelvic injury
(D) lower extremity injury

287. An injury to the spine at the level of the 6th cervical vertebra can lead to

(A) quadriplegia
(B) hemiplegia
(C) paraplegia
(D) unresponsiveness

288. The head of a patient with a suspected spinal injury should be immobilized

(A) in the neutral in-line position
(B) with the neck flexed forward
(C) with the head tilted back
(D) with the head turned to one side

289. When immobilizing a patient with suspected spinal injury, manual stabilization should be maintained until

(A) a rigid cervical collar is applied
(B) the patient's torso is secured to a spine board
(C) the patient is rolled onto a spine board
(D) the patient is completely secured to a spine board

290. The best technique for moving a supine patient onto a spine board is

(A) the four-person log roll
(B) the four-person straddle slide
(C) the two-person log roll
(D) the extremity lift

291. The most effective treatment that an EMT-Basic can give for a patient with a suspected brain injury is

(A) intravenous fluid administration
(B) ventilatory support and oxygen administration
(C) repeated suctioning
(D) application of a pneumatic antishock garment

292. Signs of brain swelling in a head-injury patient include

(A) nausea, vomiting, and confusion
(B) tachycardia and blurred vision
(C) blurred vision and hypotension
(D) tachycardia and hypotension

293. Bruising behind the ear is a sign of

(A) ear infection
(B) spinal injury
(C) skull fracture
(D) a ruptured eardrum

294. The preferred method of opening the airway in a patient with head or spinal injuries is the

(A) head-tilt/chin-lift
(B) modified jaw thrust
(C) recovery position
(D) triple airway maneuver

295. When securing a patient to a long spine board, the _____ should be secured to the board first.

(A) head
(B) cervical collar
(C) torso
(D) legs

TRAUMA

229. **The answer is B.** (AAOS, Bleeding and Shock) Elevation of an extremity with direct pressure will usually control bleeding. A tourniquet should only be used as a last resort, when all other methods of bleeding control fail. The pneumatic antishock garment will not stop bleeding from an upper extremity. Dressings, once applied, should not be removed in the field.

230. **The answer is D.** (AAOS, Bleeding and Shock) Sucking on a piece of moistened gauze may help to relieve the patient's thirst. Trauma patients should never be given anything by mouth because of the danger of vomiting and the possibility that the organs of the gastrointestinal tract are injured. Patients should never be given any alcohol.

231. **The answer is D.** (AAOS, Bleeding and Shock) As a helicopter gains altitude, the atmospheric pressure in the cabin drops. This will cause the air in the pneumatic antishock garment to expand, tightening the garment. Conversely, as the aircraft descends, the garment will loosen. The pressure must be carefully monitored and adjusted as necessary. The size of the patient and the use of immobilization equipment will not affect the pressure in the garment.

232. **The answer is D.** (Brady, Bleeding and Shock) Patients with internal bleeding usually require surgery or intensive hospital care to recover from their injuries. Internal bleeding is always serious, but it is usually not fatal if the patient receives the appropriate care in a timely manner. There is little or nothing that can be done in the field to control internal bleeding.

233. **The answer is A.** (AAOS, Bleeding and Shock) Inadequate blood flow and therefore an inadequate supply of oxygen to the organs is the cause of damage to the body by shock.

234. **The answer is D.** (AAOS, Bleeding and Shock) Once inflated, the pneumatic antishock garment should not be removed in the field. It should only be deflated gradually in the hospital after the patient has received adequate intravenous fluid replacement. Removing the garment will not help a patient whose condition has deteriorated. Removing the garment from a patient whose condition has improved or who complains of discomfort may cause a sudden drop in blood pressure.

235. **The answer is A.** (AAOS, Bleeding and Shock) Bruising on the skin of the abdomen may be a sign of internal bleeding in the abdominal cavity. This is not considered to be a minor injury. Patients with internal bleeding may develop shock, but specific signs of shock will then be present. *Melena* is dark stools that are seen when a patient has bleeding in the upper gastrointestinal tract.

236. **The answer is B.** (AAOS, Bleeding and Shock) Falling blood pressure is a sign of decompensated shock. Patients with compensated shock will maintain a normal blood pressure but will display other signs of shock such as anxiety and rapid pulse. *Hypertension* is high blood pressure. Low blood pressure is not a sign of head injury.

237. **The answer is C.** (Brady, Bleeding and Shock) The tourniquet must be proximal to the wound to be effective. It should, however, be applied as far distal as possible on the limb to limit the amount of damage it will cause. A tourniquet need not be applied over an arterial pressure point. A tourniquet located distal to the wound will have no effect on the bleeding.

238. **The answer is D.** (AAOS, Bleeding and Shock) Nosebleeds can often be controlled by pinching the nostrils together and holding them for at least 15 minutes. Nothing should ever be placed in a patient's nose. If the patient tilts the head back, blood may trickle down the throat and be inhaled into the lungs or swallowed into the stomach, where it may cause vomiting.

239. **The answer is A.** (Brady, Bleeding and Shock) Bright red blood that spurts from a wound is characteristic of arterial bleeding. Bleeding from a vein tends to produce dark maroon blood that flows steadily from the wound. Bleeding from capillaries produces a slow ooze of blood from a wound. Internal bleeding does not cause blood to appear on the surface of the body.

240. **The answer is C.** (AAOS, Bleeding and Shock) The body's normal process of coagulation will cause most wounds to stop bleeding in approximately 6 to 10 minutes.

241. **The answer is A.** (AAOS, Bleeding and Shock) Snoring is a sign of airway obstruction by the tongue. Establishing an open airway is the first priority in all critically ill patients. Use of the pneumatic antishock garment or administration of oxygen will be ineffective if the patient is breathing inadequately owing to an obstructed airway. The jaw thrust is the most appropriate initial maneuver for controlling the airway of a trauma patient, because it does not require any movement of the head and neck. The head-tilt/chin-lift should not be used for trauma patients because it involves movement of the head and neck that may aggravate spinal injuries.

242. **The answer is D.** (Brady, Bleeding and Shock) Pressure applied directly to the wound will control almost all instances of external bleeding. The pneumatic antishock garment is useful for internal bleeding from fractures of the pelvis and femur. A tourniquet should only be used as a last resort if all other methods fail. Pressure applied to arterial pressure points will slow bleeding, but will not usually control it unless used along with direct pressure.

243. **The answer is C.** (Brady, Bleeding and Shock) You should maintain pressure on the wound by securing the dressing with a bandage. This will prevent the bleeding from restarting and help to prevent infection. Removing the dressing may cause bleeding to resume. Applying a tourniquet or applying pressure to arterial pressure points is unnecessary at this point, because the bleeding has stopped.

244. **The answer is A.** (Brady, Bleeding and Shock) Elevating an extremity causes gravity to slow the flow of blood into the extremity. This will slow the bleeding and help to stop it. Direct pressure can easily be applied along with elevation. Elevation is a simple technique with few harmful effects. It should be applied routinely along with direct pressure.

245. **The answer is B.** (AAOS, Bleeding and Shock) Narrow material such as a rope, a belt, or a wire should never be used as a tourniquet because it may cut into the skin and cause serious damage to the underlying tissues. A triangular or other bandage folded into a strip 4 inches wide may be used as an effective tourniquet. A blood pressure cuff may also be used as a tourniquet if it is pumped to a pressure above the systolic blood pressure.

246. **The answer is D.** (Brady, Soft Tissue Injuries) Red blood cells are produced by the bone marrow. The skin acts as a barrier to prevent microorganisms from entering the body to cause infections. The skin helps to regulate body temperature by three mechanisms. The fat cells at the base of the skin provide insulation. The blood vessels in the skin can dilate to radiate heat outward or constrict to conserve heat. The sweat glands provide perspiration that controls the body temperature by evaporation. The skin also provides a covering that prevents the loss of water and stops external water from entering the body.

247. **The answer is B.** (Mosby, Soft Tissue Injuries) The dermis is the layer of skin below the epidermis that contains blood vessels, nerve endings, and structures such as sweat glands, sebaceous glands, and hair follicles. The epidermis is the outer layer of the skin. The surface of the epidermis that is in contact with the environment consists of dead cells that are constantly replaced by the layers beneath. The epidermis contains granules of pigment that give the skin color, but no blood vessels or nerves. The subcutaneous layer of the skin consists of fat cells that provide insulation and cushioning. Fascia is a fibrous tissue that covers muscles and joins the skin to the underlying tissue.

248. **The answer is D.** (Brady, Soft Tissue Injuries) Open wounds allow the release of blood and other body fluids. EMT-Basics must always employ the proper body substance isolation techniques prior to treating open wounds. Protective gloves should always be worn, and other items such as eye protection or gowns should be considered if there is a potential for major contamination. Once the appropriate body substance isolation techniques have been observed, the wound surface should be cleaned of major contamination. Bleeding is controlled by direct pressure, and a pressure dressing applied to the wound.

249. **The answer is B.** (AAOS, Soft Tissue Injuries) A collection of blood that can be felt as a lump under the skin at the site of a closed injury is called a *hematoma.* A *contusion* is a closed injury that results from a force being applied to body tissues. A *bruise* is a discoloration of the skin from bleeding beneath the surface. A bruise commonly results from a contusion. A bruise can be seen but not felt. A *hernia* is the protrusion of an internal organ from the cavity that normally holds it.

250. **The answer is A.** (AAOS, Soft Tissue Injuries) The abdomen of a patient with suspected internal injuries should be gently palpated for tenderness or rigidity. These are signs of internal bleeding. A fall in blood pressure is a late sign of internal bleeding. Listening for breath sounds will help to assess the condition of the lungs and chest but not the abdomen. Trauma patients should never be induced to vomit. However, if the patient vomits spontaneously, the vomitus should be examined for the presence of fresh or digested blood.

251. **The answer is C.** (Brady, Soft Tissue Injuries) Internal injuries can cause massive bleeding inside the body. Patients with suspected internal injuries should be carefully monitored for signs of shock due to blood loss. Patients with suspected internal injuries should normally be transported in the supine position. These patients should receive nothing by mouth, even if they complain of thirst, because of the danger of vomiting. The pneumatic antishock garment is useful only for certain types of internal injury, such as blood loss due to a fractured pelvis.

252. **The answer is D.** (Mosby, Soft Tissue Injuries) An injury in which a flap of skin is torn loose or completely separated from the body is known as an *avulsion.* An *abrasion* is the scraping away of the outer layers of the skin. A *laceration* is a tearing of the skin; it may be caused by a sharp object or by a severe blunt-force injury. A *puncture* is a wound that occurs when a sharp object such as a nail, icepick, or knife penetrates below the skin.

253. **The answer is C.** (Mosby, Soft Tissue Injuries) An open wound in the chest wall can admit outside air into the chest cavity and cause the lungs to collapse. An airtight dressing, also known as an *occlusive* dressing, should be applied to open chest wounds. A bulky dressing is useful to stabilize fractured ribs, but it will not stop air from entering the chest cavity. Leaving the wound open with no dressing or using a loosely applied dressing will allow air to easily enter the chest cavity.

254. **The answer is D.** (Brady, Soft Tissue Injuries) Increasing respiratory distress, shock, decreased or absent breath sounds on the side involved, tracheal deviation, and distended neck veins are signs of tension pneumothorax. If this should occur, it is necessary to lift one corner of the airtight dressing to allow the trapped air to escape. Patients with open chest

injuries should always receive the highest possible concentration of oxygen and should normally be transported in the supine position. In the absence of a suspected spinal injury, patients with a tension pneumothorax may benefit from being transported on the injured side. Raising the head of a patient with shock will decrease the flow of blood to the brain and vital organs and thus should be avoided.

255. **The answer is D.** (Brady, Soft Tissue Injuries) A patient with open or closed abdominal injuries should normally be transported lying on the back with the knees flexed to allow the abdominal muscles to relax. This will reduce pain and make the patient more comfortable. A patient in the prone position cannot be adequately monitored. The left lateral recumbent position may be useful in the absence of suspected spinal injury for patients with severe vomiting. Raising the head of a patient with potential shock will decrease the flow of blood to the brain and vital organs and should therefore be avoided.

256. **The answer is B.** (AAOS, Soft Tissue Injuries) Organs protruding from the abdominal wall should be covered with a sterile dressing that has been moistened with saline solution. This should then be covered with an air-occlusive dressing to prevent drying of the exposed organs. A bulky dry dressing will cause the loss of moisture from the exposed organs. A clean sheet will not prevent the loss of moisture and may introduce infection. Abdominal organs left exposed to the air will rapidly lose moisture.

257. **The answer is B.** (Brady, Soft Tissue Injuries) Pain, reddening, and the development of blisters are characteristic of a partial-thickness burn, also known as a *second-degree burn.* Superficial burns, also known as *first-degree burns,* present with pain, reddening, and some swelling, but no blisters. Full-thickness burns, also known as *third-degree burns,* present with an area that is charred black or brown or may appear white and dry. Full-thickness burns often destroy the nerve endings in the skin and may therefore be painless.

258. **The answer is C.** (Mosby, Soft Tissue Injuries) Using the rule of nines, the entire arm is 9 percent of the body surface area, the anterior chest is another 9 percent, and the posterior chest is another 9 percent. In this patient, therefore, a total of 27 percent of the body surface area has been burned.

259. **The answer is A.** (Mosby, Soft Tissue Injuries) Owing to the complexity of the underlying structures and the importance of the feet for weight bearing and mobility, a partial-thickness burn to the feet is considered to be critical. If there is no respiratory compromise or involvement of critical body structures such as the hands, feet, face, or genitals, a burn is considered critical if more than 10 percent of the body surface area is involved by full-thickness burns or more than 30 percent by partial-thickness burns. A partial-thickness burn of the anterior right and left legs will total 18 percent. A partial-thickness burn of the anterior chest will total 9 percent. A full-thickness burn of the anterior upper arm will be 2.25 percent.

260. The answer is A. (AAOS, Soft Tissue Injuries) Dry sterile dressings or special burn sheets are recommended for patients with extensive burns. These will help reduce the chance of infection and maintain body temperature. Wet sterile dressings are sometimes recommended for small burns covering less than 9 percent of the body surface area. Wet dressings on extensive burns can cause heat loss and hypothermia. Ointments or sprays should never be applied to a burn. They will need to be removed by painful scrubbing before the burn can be properly treated in the hospital. Air-tight dressings are not useful for burns.

261. The answer is C. (AAOS, Soft Tissue Injuries) Burns caused by caustic liquids should be flushed with large amounts of water for at least 20 minutes to remove all of the chemical from the skin. Flushing with water can continue during transport if necessary. A brief flush with water will not always remove all of the caustic liquid. That is especially true in the case of alkaline solutions. Covering a caustic liquid with a dressing will concentrate the liquid on the skin and increase the amount of damage. Chemical burns must be treated immediately in the field. Delaying treatment until arrival at a hospital will increase the amount of damage.

262. The answer is B. (Brady, Soft Tissue Injuries) Fluid and blood leaking from damaged blood vessels will cause the surrounding tissue to expand. That will be seen as swelling around the area of injury. As the injured tissue expands, pressure will be placed on nerve endings, causing the patient to feel pain. Numbness and paralysis are often signs of injury to a nerve. Burning sensations may be a sign of thermal injury.

263. The answer is D. (Brady, Musculoskeletal Injury) Pain and swelling can be seen with sprains, dislocations, or fractures. Unless there is a very gross deformity to the extremity, it is very difficult to make a precise diagnosis. Any extremity that is painful, swollen, or deformed should be immobilized with the appropriate splint.

264. The answer is D. (Brady, Musculoskeletal Injury) A painful, swollen, or deformed extremity may be the result of a fracture. Broken bone ends that are allowed to move may damage the surrounding structures and cause bleeding, pain, and nerve injury. The objective of splinting is to immobilize the extremity to prevent further injury. It is not possible to properly set bones in the field. Patients should not be allowed to walk on a painful, swollen, or deformed lower extremity.

265. The answer is A. (AAOS, Soft Tissue Injuries) The application of cold and compression along with elevation and immobilization with a splint is an effective method of controlling the bleeding and swelling seen with a closed soft tissue injury. Tourniquets are rarely necessary to control bleeding and should only be used in the most extreme cases. Pneumatic antishock garments may be used to control bleeding from fractures of the pelvis and femurs. The application of heat may make swelling worse.

266. The answer is B. (AAOS, Musculoskeletal Injury) Open injuries of this type may allow infection to begin in exposed bone ends. Infections in bone are difficult to treat and may result in loss of the limb. Patients with open musculoskeletal injuries require surgery for proper cleaning of wounds and setting of fractures. Paralysis and numbness may be signs of nerve injury. Hypothermia is not a complication of an extremity injury.

267. **The answer is A.** (AAOS, Musculoskeletal Injury) When examining an injured extremity, you may hear or feel a grating sensation that is produced when broken bones rub together. This is known as *crepitus*. Sometimes the patient has already felt the sensation and will describe it. Crepitus is often painful for the patient. You should never attempt to elicit this sensation in an injured extremity. Deformity may be observed without movement of the bone ends. The periostium is the outer covering of the bone.

268. **The answer is D.** (Brady, Musculoskeletal Injury) Injured bones may come out of alignment and cause an extremity to appear deformed or angulated. A patient may not be able to use an extremity that has suffered a musculoskeletal injury. Discoloration or bruising is often a sign of musculoskeletal injury.

269. **The answer is D.** (AAOS, Musculoskeletal Injury) The first step in treating any patient is to observe the appropriate body substance isolation techniques. This must be done prior to any assessment or treatment of the extremity. It is especially important in cases of open injury.

270. **The answer is C.** (Brady, Musculoskeletal Injury) The most important technique for treating an unstable trauma patient is rapid transport to an appropriate medical facility. Splinting each extremity individually would require a long time at the scene. Applying a traction splint properly may also take a long time. Not splinting the extremities at all would expose the patient to the possibility of further injury or disability. Splinting the patient's entire body with a long spine board will achieve acceptable immobilization in a very short time.

271. **The answer is B.** (Brady, Musculoskeletal Injury) A deformed limb should be realigned prior to splinting. Realigning a limb will help to restore and maintain circulation. It is very difficult to apply an effective splint to an extremity that is allowed to remain angulated, and there is a greater chance that an open injury will occur in a misaligned extremity. Deformity in a limb often indicates an instability of the bones, and a splint should always be applied. A pillow splint may not provide a stable enough immobilization for a deformed limb.

272. **The answer is B.** (Brady, Musculoskeletal Injury) To effectively immobilize an injured extremity, a splint must immobilize the joint above and the joint below the affected bone. If both joints are not included, the affected bone will move every time a joint that is not immobilized moves. The bone cannot be immobilized unless the adjacent joints are also immobilized.

273. **The answer is C.** (AAOS, Musculoskeletal Injury) The motion, sensation, and circulation of a painful, swollen, or deformed extremity should be assessed before and after moving or splinting the patient. It is important to know the status of the extremity prior to applying the splint. The motion, sensation, and circulation should be reassessed after the splint has been applied and periodically throughout the transport. The patient may or may not complain of numbness in cases of a nerve or blood vessel injury.

274. **The answer is B.** (AAOS, Musculoskeletal Injury) The lower leg can best be immobilized with rigid board splints. One or two boards may be used, but the splint must extend from the ankle to the knee. The pillow splint is used for ankle and foot injuries. The traction splint is used for injuries to the upper leg or thigh. The sling and swathe is used for injuries to the upper arm.

275. **The answer is D.** (AAOS, Musculoskeletal Injury) Stabilizing the airway, breathing, and circulation is always the first priority for the treatment of any trauma patient. The proper management of extremity injuries is important, but isolated limb injuries are rarely life threatening. Assessing, straightening, and splinting the patient's extremity are important, but not the first priority.

276. **The answer is C.** (AAOS, Musculoskeletal Injury) A deformed limb cannot be splinted effectively. Manual traction is applied to gently align the limb enough for a splint to be properly applied. The circulation of a limb should be assessed prior to the application of manual traction. The reducing of fractures and replacement of protruding bone ends are procedures that are done in the hospital.

277. **The answer is B.** (AAOS, Musculoskeletal Injury) After the circulation, sensation, and motor function of an extremity have been assessed, the proper way to apply manual traction is to pull gently along the long axis of the bone until the limb assumes the normal anatomic position. Traction should be stopped if there is any resistance or the patient has severe pain. The limb should never be pulled sharply or pushed in any direction away from the long axis.

278. **The answer is C.** (AAOS, Musculoskeletal Injury) The purpose of traction is to maintain the limb in the normal anatomic alignment so that bone ends do not damage adjacent structures. A limb can be further damaged if too much traction is applied. It is possible to apply excessive traction with the ratchet mechanism of the traction splint. The injured limb should never be pulled until the patient feels pain or the limb appears longer than its normal length as compared to the uninjured limb.

279. **The answer is D.** (Brady, Musculoskeletal Injury) The femur is the large bone in the thigh. If the femur is fractured, the powerful thigh muscles may contract and push the broken bone ends out of alignment. The bone ends may cause severe bleeding and damage to surrounding structures. In some cases, the bone ends are pushed through the skin, causing an open fracture. Without a traction splint, the bone ends cannot be kept in alignment against the push of the thigh muscles. The traction splint would generate too much traction

for an upper extremity. Dislocated joints should usually be splinted in the position that they are found.

280. **The answer is D.** (Brady, Musculoskeletal Injury) Injuries to the elbow often cause damage to nearby nerves and blood vessels. Elbow injuries are no more painful than injuries to other joints, and they can be splinted easily with a moldable splint. There is not enough space in the elbow joint to allow life-threatening bleeding. The patient's distal circulation, sensation, and motor function should be assessed often when dealing with an elbow injury.

281. **The answer is B.** (AAOS, Musculoskeletal Injury) Injuries to the hand can result in severe disability if they are not handled correctly. A roller gauze or bulky dressing should be placed in the palm of the injured hand, and the hand formed around it with the fingers slightly flexed. Splinting the hand in the flat or clenched position may aggravate the patient's injuries. Traction splints are not used for upper extremity injuries.

282. **The answer is C.** (AAOS, Musculoskeletal Injury) The pelvis has a very rich blood supply, and many large blood vessels are located near the pelvis. Injuries to the pelvis can cause severe internal bleeding that can be life threatening. Patients with pelvic injuries should be monitored carefully for the presence of shock. Pelvic injuries are also associated with damage to the urinary bladder and with disability, but these problems are not life threatening.

283. **The answer is C.** (Brady, Musculoskeletal Injury) This patient has a pelvic injury with signs of shock. The pneumatic antishock garment (PASG) should be applied, and all compartments inflated. The PASG will provide immobilization and pressure on any internal bleeding that may be the cause of the shock. A long spine board will provide some immobilization, but not pressure on bleeding vessels. Rigid splints and traction splints cannot be used on the pelvis.

284. **The answer is C.** (AAOS, Musculoskeletal Injury) In most cases, a joint should be splinted in the position in which it is found. Leaving an injured joint without a splint may lead to further injury. However, if the limb is pulseless, there is a chance that there may be severe, permanent damage to the limb if circulation is not restored quickly. One attempt should be made to realign the knee and restore the distal circulation. Traction splints should not be applied to an injured knee.

285. **The answer is D.** (Mosby, Musculoskeletal Injury) An effective splint for an injured foot can be made by wrapping a pillow around the foot and securing it with cravats. The pillow will cushion and elevate the foot while providing immobilization. The pillow will not provide sufficient support to splint the lower leg or upper arm. The hand should be splinted in the position of function by use of a bulky dressing.

286. **The answer is B.** (AAOS, Injuries to the Head and Spine) An unconscious trauma victim must always be presumed to have a spinal injury. A spinal injury that is not properly immobilized can lead to paralysis or death. All unconscious trauma victims should be immobilized with a cervical collar and spine board. The EMT-Basic should suspect internal bleeding, pelvic injury, or lower extremity injury on the basis of the mechanism of injury and physical findings.

287. **The answer is A.** (AAOS, Injuries to the Head and Spine) An injury at the level of the 6th cervical vertebra in the neck may cause *quadriplegia,* which is paralysis of all four limbs. Injuries lower down on the spine can cause paralysis in the lower extremities, known as *paraplegia. Hemiplegia* is paralysis on one side of the body; it is seen in patients with a stroke. Unresponsiveness is seen mostly with head injuries.

288. **The answer is A.** (AAOS, Injuries to the Head and Spine) The head of a patient with a spinal injury should be carefully moved to the neutral in-line position (also known as the eyes-forward position). Moving the head to this position will make immobilization easier and more effective. Flexing, tilting, or turning the patient's head may aggravate a spinal injury.

289. **The answer is D.** (Brady, Injuries to the Head and Spine) Manual stabilization should be maintained until a patient is completely secured to a spine board. A rigid cervical collar provides some degree of support, but the cervical spine can still move with a cervical collar in place. When a patient has been partially secured to the spine board, there can still be movement of the cervical spine.

290. **The answer is A.** (AAOS, Injuries to the Head and Spine) The four-person log roll provides the most support and causes the least movement to a patient with an injured spine. The four-person straddle slide is useful when there is no access to the side of the patient, but it does not provide as much support as the log roll. The log roll can be performed by two persons, but there will be more movement than with four persons. Lifting of a spinal injury patient should be avoided.

291. **The answer is B.** (AAOS, Injuries to the Head and Spine) The amount of swelling to the brain of a head injury patient can be reduced by making sure that the patient is well ventilated and well oxygenated. Head-injury patients should receive high-concentration oxygen even if there is no sign of respiratory distress. Repeated suctioning may cause hypoxia. EMT-Basics do not administer intravenous fluids. The pneumatic antishock garment is not helpful for head-injury patients.

292. **The answer is A.** (AAOS, Injuries to the Head and Spine) Patients with swelling of the brain due to head injury become confused and suffer nausea and vomiting. If the swelling progresses, the blood pressure will rise and the pulse rate will fall.

293. **The answer is C.** (AAOS, Injuries to the Head and Spine) Bruising behind the ear, known as *Battle's sign,* is a sign of a basal skull fracture. Patients with this type of injury often have bilateral black eyes, known as *raccoon eyes.* Blood or clear fluid may also be seen draining from the ears, the nose, or around the eyes of a patient with this type of injury.

294. **The answer is B.** (AAOS, Injuries to the Head and Spine) The modified jaw thrust will cause the least amount of movement to the head and neck when opening the airway. The head can be maintained in the neutral in-line position while applying the modified jaw thrust. The head-tilt/ chin-lift, recovery position, and triple airway maneuver cause significant movement of the head.

295. **The answer is C.** (Brady, Injuries to the Head and Spine) In order to minimize movement of the cervical spine, the patient's torso should be secured to the spine board first. Once the torso has been secured with belts, the head can be secured with a commercial or improvised head immobilization device. The cervical collar is not normally secured to the spine board.

INFANTS AND CHILDREN

Directions: Each item below contains four suggested responses. Select the **one best** response to each item.

296. All of the following are developmental characteristics of newborns and infants (birth to 1 year) EXCEPT that

(A) there is minimal stranger anxiety
(B) they are used to being undressed, but like to be warm
(C) they do not like to be separated from their parents
(D) they readily accept an oxygen mask

297. All of the following are developmental characteristics of toddlers (ages 1 to 3 years) EXCEPT that

(A) they are comfortable with being undressed
(B) they do not like to be touched or separated from their parents
(C) they have a fear of needles and pain
(D) they do not like being suffocated by an oxygen mask

298. All of the following are developmental characteristics of preschool children (3 to 6 years) EXCEPT that

(A) they are modest and do not want their clothing removed
(B) they have a fear of blood, pain, and permanent injury
(C) they are not curious, are very quiet, and will rarely cooperate
(D) they do not want to be suffocated by an oxygen mask

299. All of the following are developmental characteristics of school-age children (6 to 12 years) EXCEPT that

(A) they cooperate but like their opinions heard
(B) they are modest and do not like to expose their bodies
(C) they do not want to be suffocated by an oxygen mask
(D) they fear blood, pain, disfigurement, and permanent injury

300. All of the following are developmental characteristics of adolescent children (12 to 18 years) EXCEPT that

(A) they often need to be physically restrained because of inappropriate fears of treatment
(B) they want to be treated as adults
(C) they often feel that they are indestructible, but they may fear permanent injury and disfigurement
(D) they may not be comfortable exposing their changing bodies

301. All of the following are age-specific responses to illness or injury, EXCEPT that

(A) newborns and infants (birth to age 1 year) are usually frightened by strangers
(B) toddlers (age 1 to 3 years) are afraid if they are in pain or bleeding and need reassurance
(C) preschool children (age 3 to 6 years) have active imaginations and may invent strange and frightening ideas about what is happening
(D) school-age children (age 6 to 12 years) fear pain, blood, and permanent injury

302. In comparing the anatomy of infants and children with that of an adult, all of the following are true EXCEPT that

(A) the most important anatomic and physiologic differences in infants and children relate to the heart
(B) in infants and children, the airways are smaller and more easily blocked by secretions and/or swollen tissues
(C) in opening the airway in infants and children, if you hyperextend the neck, you may actually occlude the flexible airway
(D) in infants and children, the tongue is relatively large in relation to the small mandible and oropharynx. This may cause airway obstruction in the unresponsive, supine infant or child

303. All of the following are causes of pediatric respiratory emergencies EXCEPT

(A) partial and complete airway obstruction
(B) croup
(C) epiglottitis
(D) congestive heart failure

304. You are dispatched to a "child with dif-ficulty breathing" and find a 3-year-old boy who appears sick. The child's mother tells you that he has had a fever, a barking cough, and increasing diffi-culty breathing. The most likely cause of this infectious illness is croup or epiglottitis. In assessing and treating this child, the most important thing to avoid is

(A) mentioning the possible cause of the illness
(B) administering cool-mist blow-by oxygen
(C) allowing the child to be trans-ported sitting in his parent's lap
(D) inserting a finger, tongue blade, or oral airway into the child's mouth

305. You respond to the scene of an uncon-scious 5-year-old girl. The girl's hysteri-cal mother said that her daughter was running around the house with a piece of hot dog in her mouth. She suddenly stopped running and grabbed for her throat and stopped talking. Within a short period, she collapsed, passed out, and stopped breathing. The best descrip-tion of this type of pediatric respiratory emergency is

(A) acute croup or epiglottitis
(B) complete airway obstruction due to a foreign body
(C) an anaphylactic reaction
(D) incomplete airway obstruction due to a foreign body

306. You are dispatched to a child with difficulty breathing and arrive to find a 3-year-old child who is in respiratory distress, breathing 40 times per minute. The child's mother states that they were having a birthday party when she noticed that this child was running around with a toy balloon in his mouth. Suddenly, he stopped and began to have difficulty breathing and became frightened. Your assessment shows that he is awake, with noisy respirations and use of accessory muscles. All of the following are appro-priate in delivering emergency care to this child with a partial airway obstruc-tion EXCEPT to

(A) encourage the child to sit up, in a position of comfort (often in a parent's lap)
(B) administer oxygen by the blow-by method
(C) secure the child to the parent's lap for transport by buckling a lap belt over both
(D) make every effort to keep the child comfortable and nonagitated

307. You are dispatched to an infant with respiratory distress. As you drive up to the house, the mother is running towards you with her 6-month-old baby who is in respiratory distress—tachypneic, with marked retractions, and cyanotic. The mother notes that small pieces of her other child's toys were found in this infant's crib. While quickly assessing this awake infant, you note that the baby is unable to cry or cough as well. Which of the following is the best method of providing emergency care to this infant?

(A) Immediately lie the child supine on the ground and only administer blow-by oxygen

(B) Immediately perform a blind finger sweep to try to feel a foreign body and remove it

(C) Immediately begin a series of five abdominal thrusts (Heimlich maneuver), using a fisted hand, between the umbilicus and the xiphoid

(D) With proper support to the infant, rapidly alternate five back blows and five chest thrusts until the obstruction is relieved or the child becomes unresponsive

308. All of the following are signs of respiratory distress EXCEPT

(A) increased respiratory rate

(B) wheezing

(C) use of accessory muscles (intercostal and supraclavicular retractions)

(D) cyanosis

309. All of the following are signs of respiratory failure EXCEPT

(A) a respiratory rate of over 60 or under 20 breaths per minute

(B) severe retractions

(C) cyanosis

(D) increased muscle tone

310. You are dispatched to a child in respiratory distress. As you arrive in the child's apartment, you find a frightened 6-year-old boy who is breathing 44 times per minute. His mother says that he has had a cold and has been wheezing for a few days. Which of the following is the correct emergency care for this child?

(A) Encourage the child to lie down, with a tight oxygen face mask

(B) Allow the child to sit up, administer oxygen by a loose-fitting face mask, and transport to the hospital

(C) Allow the child to sit up and administer your beta-agonist albuterol inhaler

(D) Apply a tight bag-valve-mask device and assist ventilations right away

311. While you are riding in your assigned ambulance district you are waved down by a woman who states that her daughter is having severe difficulty breathing. While walking up to the woman's apartment, she tells you that her 8-year-old daughter has had a high fever, sore throat, and productive cough with yellow phlegm for 4 days. Upon assessing the child, you find an 8-year-old girl, drowsy, breathing at 12 times per minute, with severe retractions, severe accessory muscle use, and cyanosis. The correct emergency care for this child is to

(A) have her sit up and to administer blow-by oxygen
(B) try to administer a beta-agonist bronchodilator oral inhaler
(C) transport her sitting up in her parent's lap without any prior assistance
(D) place the child supine on a stretcher, and assist the ventilations with high-concentration oxygen via a bag-valve-mask device

312. All of the following are signs of shock in infants and children EXCEPT

(A) a rapid heartbeat
(B) pale, cool, clammy skin
(C) strong peripheral pulses
(D) an altered level of consciousness

313. You are dispatched to a "sick child". You arrive at the child's apartment to find a limp 3-year-old lying in his mother's arms. The mother states that the child has been vomiting with diarrhea for two days now. In this 3-year-old child in shock, all of the following would be consistent with poor end-organ perfusion EXCEPT

(A) delayed capillary refill (greater than 2 seconds)
(B) tachycardia
(C) weak or absent peripheral pulses
(D) full alertness

314. The usual cause of nontraumatic cardiac arrest in the adult is a cardiac disorder (arrhythmia, acute myocardial infarction, congestive heart failure, etc.). In infants and children, the usual cause of nontraumatic cardiac arrest is

(A) cardiac disease
(B) respiratory disease
(C) poisoning
(D) status epilepticus

315. All of the following are causes of seizures in infants and children EXCEPT

(A) leg injury
(B) chronic seizure disorder
(C) head trauma
(D) fever

316. You are dispatched to the scene of a 2-year-old girl with "seizures". When you arrive at the child's home, her father tells you that the child has had a fever, up to 104° F, for the past two days. Then, about 15 minutes ago, the girl began shaking violently for 5 minutes, then stopped. The child's father demonstrates tonic-clonic contractions, just as the child begins to have a second seizure. All of the following are parts of the emergency care of infants and children with seizures EXCEPT

(A) opening and maintaining the airway
(B) inserting an oropharyngeal airway during the seizure
(C) if there is no risk of spinal injury, positioning the patient on one side
(D) providing oxygen

317. Injury patterns are different in infants and children from those of adults. All of the following are accurate descriptions of such similarities or differences EXCEPT

(A) musculoskeletal trauma is the same in infants and children as in adults
(B) because of the smaller size of infants and children, traumatic forces spread throughout the body, rather than over a small area
(C) because the internal organs of infants and children are small and close together, more energy is transmitted to more organs by a given injury than for an adult
(D) there may be more serious internal damage without serious outward signs in infants and children than in adults

318. Which of the following is the most common cause of death in pediatric trauma patients?

(A) Chest injury
(B) Abdominal injury
(C) Head injury
(D) Burns

319. You are dispatched to the scene of a motor vehicle accident. At the scene, there is a screaming mother, who states that she skidded and hit the back door of her car on a telephone pole. She screams that her 3-year-old daughter is in her car seat in the back of the car. Your assessment reveals a 3-year-old girl who is unconscious in her car seat. Which of the following is the correct sequence for providing emergency care to this child?

(A) Carefully remove the child from the car seat and immediately transport her in her mother's arms
(B) Quickly remove the child from the car seat and immediately transport her in one of the EMT's arms
(C) Apply a tight-fitting oxygen mask and leave the child unconscious in her car seat
(D) Open the child's airway first, using the jaw-thrust maneuver, then immobilize the child in the car seat

320. You are dispatched to the scene of a child who fell down a flight of stairs. Upon arrival, you find a 7-year-old boy at the bottom of the stairs. He is responsive but complains of severe chest pain from having landed on an umbrella stand with his chest. All of the following are correct elements of the emergency care of a child with chest injuries EXCEPT

(A) performing rapid assessment
(B) confirming the airway and ventilating with oxygen
(C) providing rapid transport
(D) performing spinal immobilization only if there are specific indicators of spinal injury

321. All of the following are signs of child abuse EXCEPT

(A) repeated calls for a child's injury to the same address
(B) a child who has multiple injuries at different stages of healing
(C) a smiling child who openly discusses the injury
(D) a child with fresh burns

322. You arrive at the scene of a 4-year-old child who has possibly "broken his leg". As you approach the child, you find a quiet, withdrawn 4-year-old with a swollen, very tender left calf. Upon further inspection, you find finger prints across his right cheek. His back reveals two areas of scarring. The child's father states that the boy is "very prone to injury", but no one knows exactly what happened to cause today's injury. You suspect child abuse. For an EMT-Basic all of the following are correct approaches to dealing with this possibility EXCEPT to

(A) try to discuss this possibility openly with the parents and child at the scene
(B) maintain a calm, professional manner, treat the child's injuries, and encourage transport to the hospital
(C) be familiar with the state, regional, and city laws governing the reporting of child abuse
(D) carefully document the history and physical findings of the case, and make the physician at the hospital aware of the findings and the suspicion of child abuse

323. You are dispatched to the scene of a "child struck by a car". Upon arrival, you find a 5-year-old girl, who ran into the street after a ball. A witness states that the child was hit and thrown 20 feet and upon impact hit her head on another parked car. Your initial assessment reveals a 5-year-old girl who is unconscious and not breathing, has no pulse, and has a deep open head wound. You provide all of the appropriate emergency care, including opening the airway with a jaw thrust maneuver, ventilating the patient, full spinal immobilization, proper wound care, and rapid transport to the hospital, but the child dies in the emergency department. While assisting with the care in the emergency department and immediately after the child is pronounced dead, you begin to feel very upset, anxious, and tearful. Which of the following is the best way to try to deal with your reaction to this difficult call?

(A) Try to calm down, gather your equipment, and head back on duty right away
(B) Seek out your supervisor and/or medical director to discuss the case and your reactions and feelings (debriefing)
(C) Discuss the case briefly with your partner and return to duty immediately
(D) Call your department and state that you are sick and need to go home, without discussing the case

INFANTS AND CHILDREN

296. The answer is D. (AAOS, Infant and Child Emergency Care) Choices A, B, and C are all correct. Also, younger infants follow movement with their eyes; older infants are more active, developing a personality. Choice D is incorrect because infants do not want to be suffocated by an oxygen mask.

297. The answer is A. (AAOS, Infant and Child Emergency Care) Choices B, C, and D are all correct. Toddlers also frighten easily, begin to assert their independence, and may believe that their illness is a punishment for being bad. Choice A is incorrect because toddlers do not like having their clothes removed.

298. The answer is C. (AAOS, Infant and Child Emergency Care) Choices A, B, and D are all correct. Preschoolers also do not like to be touched or separated from their parents. They also may believe that their illness is a punishment for being bad. Choice C is incorrect; preschoolers are usually curious and communicative, and they may be cooperative.

299. The answer is C. (AAOS, Infant and Child Emergency Care) School-age children will often accept an oxygen mask, if you take the time to explain its use.

300. The answer is A. (AAOS, Infant and Child Emergency Care) Adolescents do not require physical restraints for emergency care treatment. However, while they prefer to be treated as adults, they often need as much support and reassurance as children.

301. The answer is A. (AAOS, Infant and Child Emergency Care) Newborns and infants are usually not frightened by strangers. The other choices are true. Adolescents (age 12 to 18) are very concerned about permanent injury and how they will look as a result.

302. The answer is A. (Mosby, Infant and Child Emergency Care) The most important anatomic and physiologic differences in infants and children, compared to adults, is with the airway.

303. The answer is D. (AAOS, Infant and Child Emergency Care) Congestive heart failure is a pediatric *cardiac* emergency, not a respiratory emergency, even though the child presents with respiratory distress.

304. The answer is D. (AAOS, Infant and Child Emergency Care) Inserting a finger, tongue blade, or oral airway into this child's mouth could cause increased swelling and total obstruction of the airway. Choices A through C all describe reasonable assessment and treatment approaches for the child with acute respiratory distress due to croup or epiglottitis.

305. The answer is B. (AAOS, Infant and Child Emergency Care) B is the correct answer because, while running with a piece of hot dog in her mouth, this 5-year-old girl developed complete airway obstruction manifested by sudden inability to speak, became unconscious and stopped breathing. Acute croup or epiglottitis is an infectious illness manifested by fever, hoarseness, stridor, and noisy breathing. It may result in partial or complete airway obstruction. An anaphylactic reaction, while it may result in complete airway obstruction, is the result of an allergic reaction, for example, to penicillin, a bee sting, sesame seeds, etc. An incomplete airway obstruction would leave the child awake, alert, able to speak, and able to breathe.

306. The answer is C. (Brady, Infant and Child Emergency Care) In transport, you should never buckle a lap belt over both the child and parent. Choices A, B and D are true. In addition if the child demonstrates a change in color, cyanosis, or mental status deterioration, a complete obstruction has probably occurred.

307. The answer is D. (Brady, Infant and Child Emergency Care) This is the correct emergency care for a responsive infant with a foreign body airway obstruction who is unable to cry or cough effectively. A is incorrect because you need to aggressively attempt to relieve the foreign body airway obstruction before the child becomes unconscious and/or stops breathing. B is incorrect because finger sweeps are only performed in unresponsive infants after a series of five back blows and five chest thrusts, after opening the mouth with a tongue jaw lift, and only if you visualize a foreign body. You never perform a blind finger sweep. C is incorrect because abdominal thrusts are not used in infants to relieve foreign body airway obstruction.

308. The answer is D. (Brady, Infant and Child Emergency Care) Cyanosis is usually a sign of respiratory failure, not respiratory distress. The signs in choices A through C are correct. In addition, nasal flaring, mottled skin color, use of abdominal muscles, see-saw respirations, stridor, and grunting are also signs of respiratory distress.

309. The answer is D. (Brady, Infant and Child Emergency Care) The child with respiratory failure has decreased, not increased, muscle tone. The signs in choices A through C are all correct. In addition, altered mental status, severe use of accessory muscles, decreased muscle tone, and poor peripheral perfusion are also signs of respiratory failure.

310. **The answer is B.** (AAOS, Infant and Child Emergency Care) If the child develops cyanosis, then you will need to assist the ventilations. A is incorrect, because you want to encourage the child to sit up in his position of comfort and allow oxygen to be administered comfortably by an oxygen mask. C is incorrect, because you may only assist a known asthmatic to administer his or her own oral inhaler. As an EMT-Basic, you must not initiate a new oral beta-agonist bronchodilator inhaler. D is incorrect, because you only assist ventilations with a bag-valve-mask device if the child develops cyanosis.

311. **The answer is D.** (Brady, Infant and Child Emergency Care) This is the correct emergency care for a child with respiratory failure. A is incorrect; to have the child sit up and administer oxygen is the correct emergency care for a child with respiratory distress, not with respiratory failure. B is incorrect because you can only administer an inhaler that has already been prescribed by the child's physician. C is incorrect because a child with respiratory failure requires active emergency care immediately, to prevent worsening of the condition and eventual respiratory arrest.

312. **The answer is C.** (AAOS, Infant and Child Emergency Care) A, B, and D are all signs of shock in infants and children. Delayed capillary refill (longer than 2 seconds), decreased urinary output, and a decreased ability to form tears are also signs of shock in infants and children. C is incorrect because infants and children in shock have weak or absent peripheral pulses.

313. **The answer is D.** (Brady, Infant and Child Emergency Care) A, B, and C are all signs of poor end-organ perfusion due to shock. D is incorrect because the child in shock would have decreased cerebral perfusion, which may produce an altered mental status, manifested by agitation, disorientation, or unresponsiveness.

314. **The answer is B.** (Brady, Infant and Child Emergency Care) Because respiratory disease is the most common cause of nontraumatic respiratory arrest, it is important to always open and maintain the airway. A, C, and D represent less likely causes of nontraumatic cardiac arrest in infants and children.

315. **The answer is A.** (Mosby, Infant and Child Emergency Care) In addition to the ones listed in B through D, infections, poisoning, low blood sugar, low levels of oxygen, chronic medical conditions, and unknown reasons are all causes of seizures in infants and children. A leg injury is not a cause of seizures.

316. **The answer is B.** (Mosby, Infant and Child Emergency Care) In addition to the measures listed in A, C, and D, having suction available for vomiting, and transport are all correct parts of the emergency care for the seizing infant and child. Also, if the seizure lasts more than 5 to 10 minutes, or if repeated seizures occur, consider calling for ALS backup to deliver antiseizure medications.

317. The answer is A. (Mosby, Infant and Child Emergency Care) Children's bones are less calcified and more resilient than those of adults, which makes the musculoskeletal system less likely to absorb the impact of trauma.

318. The answer is C. (Mosby, Infant and Child Emergency Care) A, B, and D represent frequent causes of pediatric trauma and death, but not the most common cause.

319. The answer is D. (Mosby, Infant and Child Emergency Care) D gives the correct emergency care for a child who is unconscious owing to a traumatic injury and who may have a spinal injury. A and B are incorrect because to remove an unconscious child involved in a motor vehicle accident from a car seat without taking spinal precautions truly risks producing or aggravating a spinal injury. C is incorrect because this unconscious child requires careful jaw-thrust opening of the airway and spinal immobilization before oxygen is administered.

320. The answer is D. (Mosby, Infant and Child Emergency Care) In addition to the measures in A through C, spinal immobilization, being ready to suction if vomiting begins, and careful monitoring of vital signs are all parts of emergency care provided to a child with chest injuries. D is incorrect because a child with a possible serious chest injury due to falling down a flight of stairs always requires spinal immobilization.

321. The answer is C. (AAOS, Infant and Child Emergency Care) An abused child often appears withdrawn, fearful, and hostile and usually refuses to discuss how the injury occurred.

322. The answer is A. (AAOS, Infant and Child Emergency Care) The EMT-Basic should not accuse the parents or others of child abuse. This is obviously a highly emotionally charged subject and may impede assisting the child. It may also actually delay having the proper authorities investigate the case and be able to act on the findings.

323. The answer is B. (AAOS, Infant and Child Emergency Care) Debriefing will allow you to openly discuss the stress and extremely emotionally upsetting nature of this call. It will also allow your supervisor to discuss other options available to help you deal with this situation. None of the other choices allows you the needed opportunity to discuss the case and your reaction to it.

OPERATIONS

Directions: Each item below contains four suggested responses. Select the **one best** response to each item.

324. Ambulances should be equipped with a suction unit capable of providing a vacuum of _____ mm Hg when the tubing is clamped.

(A) 100
(B) 200
(C) 300
(D) 400

325. When responding with lights and siren on a multilane highway, the emergency vehicle operator should

(A) travel in the right lane
(B) travel down the center of the roadway
(C) travel in the left lane
(D) move from lane to lane to pass slow-moving traffic

326. The largest source of legal actions against EMS operators is

(A) medical malpractice
(B) slander and libel accusations
(C) motor vehicle accidents
(D) assault and battery complaints

327. An emergency vehicle should never

(A) exceed the posted speed limits
(B) proceed through a red signal
(C) drive against the flow of traffic
(D) pass a stopped schools bus that is displaying its flashing red lights

328. An ambulance should have a police escort

    (A) if the ambulance operator is unfamiliar with the area

    (B) to move more quickly than traffic

    (C) to ensure that other motorists yield the right of way

    (D) whenever transporting a critical patient

329. EMT-Basics should make use of which of the following types of equipment on every run?

    (A) Emergency warning lights

    (B) A siren or other audible warning device

    (C) Protective turnout gear

    (D) Seatbelts

330. A medical evacuation helicopter should always be approached

    (A) from the front

    (B) from the rear

    (C) from the side

    (D) after the rotor stops turning

331. A helicopter landing zone should be

    (A) a level area 100 feet by 100 feet

    (B) a sloping area 50 feet by 100 feet

    (C) a level area 50 feet by 50 feet

    (D) at least 200 feet by 200 feet

332. Ambulances are most likely to be involved in accidents

    (A) during inclement weather

    (B) at intersections

    (C) when traveling on limited-access highways

    (D) when traveling in reverse

333. Before entering an intersection, an emergency vehicle operator should

    (A) speed up so as to clear the intersection quickly

    (B) slow down and be prepared to stop if the way is not clear

    (C) move to the far right lane

    (D) travel at a steady speed while sounding the siren

334. The first step in attempting to gain access to a patient who is in a wrecked automobile is to

    (A) break the window farthest from the patient and crawl in

    (B) pry open the door nearest the patient

    (C) try to open the doors in the normal manner

    (D) pry out the windshield

335. The initial assessment and treatment of a patient who is trapped in an auto should be conducted

    (A) while the patient is still trapped in the auto

    (B) only after the patient has been extricated from the auto

    (C) only en route to the hospital

    (D) after the vehicle roof has been removed

336. The staging sector at a multiple-casualty incident is responsible for

(A) sorting and prioritizing patients according to severity of injury
(B) organizing arriving resources and assigning tasks
(C) removing victims from any danger or entrapment
(D) acquiring sufficient equipment and supplies

337. At the scene of a multiple-casualty incident, a patient with an isolated fracture of the wrist should be assigned a

(A) red tag
(B) yellow tag
(C) green tag
(D) black tag

338. The first EMS unit arriving at the scene of a multiple casualty incident should

(A) begin to treat the most seriously injured patients
(B) begin to triage the patients at the scene
(C) transport the most seriously injured patients
(D) retreat from the scene and await the arrival of additional resources

OPERATIONS

324. The answer is C. (Brady, Ambulance Operations) Ambulances should be equipped with portable and installed suction units. These units should be able to provide a vacuum of 300 mm Hg. The amount of vacuum must be controllable for use on infants and children.

325. The answer is C. (AAOS, Ambulance Operations) The best strategy for an emergency vehicle operator is to travel in the left lane. This will allow motorists to move to the right and allow the emergency vehicle to pass. Frequent lane changes and traveling on the right or center should be avoided, because motorists may become confused and move into the path of the emergency vehicle.

326. The answer is C. (AAOS, Ambulance Operations) Motor vehicle accidents are the most common cause of legal action against EMS operators. While every state grants right-of-way privileges to emergency vehicles, operators may be held liable if they operate their vehicles without due regard for the other motorists and pedestrians on the road.

327. The answer is D. (Brady, Ambulance Operations) An emergency vehicle operator should never pass a school bus that is stopped and displaying its flashing red lights. This indicates that the bus is loading or discharging children. The emergency vehicle operator must stop and wait for the bus driver to signal that all of the children are safe before proceeding. Emergency vehicles are generally exempt from all regulations regarding posted speed limits, traffic signals, and traffic flow. However, the operator must always use due regard for the safety of others.

328. The answer is A. (Brady, Ambulance Operations) The use of police escorts is very dangerous. In most instances, a single emergency vehicle can move more safely and quickly than two vehicles in tandem. Motorists hearing sirens may assume that the police car is the only emergency vehicle, and consequently may proceed after the police car has passed and collide with the ambulance. The only reason for an ambulance to have an escort is when the operator is unfamiliar with the area. The escorting police car serves to guide the ambulance to the scene or to the hospital.

329. The answer is D. (Brady, Ambulance Operations) Seatbelts should be worn by EMT-Basics on every run. The only exception is when the EMT-Basic is engaged in patient care that cannot be performed while wearing a seatbelt. Emergency warning lights, sirens, and protective clothing should be used as necessary.

330. The answer is A. (AAOS, Ambulance Operations) Helicopters should always be approached from the front. EMT-Basics should only proceed when the pilot signals that it is safe to do so. The pilot may not see anyone who approaches from the side of the aircraft. If the pilot does not stop the engine, be sure that you will clear the aircraft's rotor, and secure any loose items that may be blown around or sucked into the aircraft's intake. Approaching a helicopter from the rear is especially dangerous, because the rapidly spinning tail rotor may not be readily visible.

331. The answer is A. (Brady, Ambulance Operations) Whenever possible, a helicopter landing zone should be an area at least 100 feet by 100 feet square. The area should also be as level as possible, with a slope of no more than 10 degrees. This will ensure that the pilot has sufficient area to land safely with adequate clearance for the aircraft rotors.

332. The answer is B. (AAOS, Ambulance Operations) Ambulances are most likely to be involved in an accident when proceeding through an intersection. Other motorists may not see or yield to an ambulance at an intersection. The next most common type of accident occurs when an ambulance is traveling in reverse. Accidents on limited-access highways and weather-related accidents are less common.

333. The answer is B. (AAOS, Ambulance Operations) When approaching an intersection, an emergency vehicle operator must be prepared for motorists that may not yield the right of way. The emergency vehicle operator should slow down enough to be able to stop the vehicle if the intersection is not clear. An emergency vehicle operator must never assume that lights and sirens will guarantee that other motorists will yield the right of way. Speeding up will increase the severity of any collision that occurs.

334. The answer is C. (AAOS, Scene Techniques) Always try the safest and simplest solution first. Even though an automobile may be seriously damaged, one or more of the doors may operate in the normal manner. Try all of the doors before taking any other steps. If none of the doors will open, carefully break the window farthest from the patient and crawl through the opening. Removing a windshield or forcing a door requires special training and equipment.

335. The answer is A. (AAOS, Scene Techniques) Unless there is a dangerous situation, the initial assessment and treatment of a patient who is trapped in an automobile should be conducted while the patient is still trapped in the auto. Automobile extrications may take a long time on the scene. Life-threatening conditions may be identified and treated as the extrication is in process. This approach will help to ensure that the patient receives treatment and transport in a timely fashion.

336. The answer is B. (AAOS, Scene Techniques) Arriving resources at a multiple-casualty incident report to the staging sector to be organized and to receive their assignments. Victims are removed from danger or entrapment by the extrication sector and then brought to the triage sector for sorting and prioritizing. The supply sector is responsible for acquiring equipment and supplies that may be required at the scene.

337. The answer is C. (AAOS, Scene Techniques) It is possible to delay the treatment and transport of a patient with a single isolated injury such as a fractured wrist. This patient should receive a green tag. Patients with life-threatening injuries or illnesses that need immediate treatment and transport should receive a red tag. Patients with moderately severe or multiple injuries are considered second priority and receive a yellow tag. Patients who are not breathing or have obvious mortal injuries are the lowest priority and should receive a black tag.

338. The answer is B. (AAOS, Scene Techniques) The first arriving unit should immediately size up the scene and begin to triage patients. At the scene of a multiple-casualty incident, it is of primary importance to sort the patients in accordance with the severity of their condition. Further arriving units can begin treatment in accordance with the triage priorities established by first arriving unit. Transport is begun after the patients have been triaged and treatment has begun.

ADVANCED AIRWAY

Directions: Each item below contains four suggested responses. Select the **one best** response to each item.

339. The three areas of the airway labeled on the diagram are anatomically different in the child than in the adult in ways that are important for airway management. These areas are

(A) 1) the palate; 2) the uvula;
3) the esophagus

(B) 1) the oropharynx; 2) the tonsils;
3) the bronchus

(C) 1) the tongue; 2) the glottis;
3) the cricoid area

(D) 1) the glottis; 2) the hyoid;
3) the pharynx

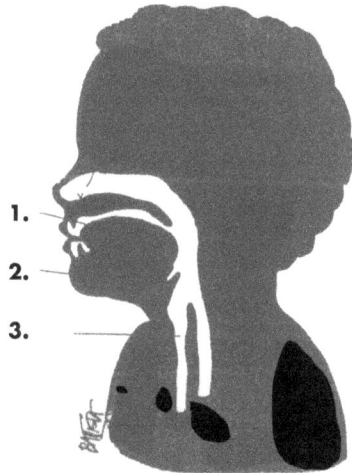

1.

2.

3.

340. All of the following are true statements concerning the anatomy of the infant, child, and adult airways EXCEPT that

(A) in infants and children, the tongue takes up more space in the mouth than in the adult

(B) the cricoid ring is the narrowest portion of the airway in infants and children

(C) the size of the head relative to the body is the same in infants, children, and adults

(D) the trachea and vocal cords in children are higher and lie more anteriorly than in the adult

341. All of the following are means by which the airway can become compromised EXCEPT that

(A) in the unconscious adult, the person's own teeth can slip back to block the airway

(B) when infants and children lie on their backs, the head is forced into a flexed position and can compromise the airway

(C) a child's tongue takes up more space in the mouth than adult's tongue; therefore, in a child, it is even more important to open the airway by lifting the tongue

(D) the smaller diameter of the airway in infants and children increases the chance of airway obstruction by small items, fluid, or swelling

342. All of the following statements regarding airway adjuncts (oropharyngeal and nasopharyngeal airways) are true EXCEPT that

(A) other names for the oropharyngeal airway are the *oral airway* and the *OP airway*

(B) in the unconscious patient with a positive gag reflex, the oropharyngeal airway can be inserted carefully

(C) the method for inserting the oral airway is different for adults than for children

(D) the nasopharyngeal airways (also called the *nasal airway* or *NP airway*) is inserted in the same manner for adults and children and is the best airway adjunct for the seizing patient

343. All of the following statements are true about the use of oxygen therapy in the emergently ill patient EXCEPT that

(A) the preferred method for delivering oxygen in the prehospital setting is by a nonrebreather mask. When set at 15 liters per minute, this device can deliver 90 percent oxygen to the patient

(B) a patient who is uncomfortable with a tight mask on the face may be allowed to hold the mask on the face

(C) the delivery of high-concentration oxygen is indicated for any patient who complains of difficulty breathing, is cyanotic, or has cool, clammy skin

(D) nonrebreather masks should fit from the bridge of the nose to just below the chin

344. Nasogastric tubes are used to decompress the stomach and the proximal bowel of air. All of the following are true statements about nasogastric tubes EXCEPT that

(A) the primary indication for the use of the nasogastric tubes in the prehospital setting is an inability to artificially ventilate an infant or child because of gastric distention

(B) the equipment used during insertion of the nasogastric tube includes a water-soluble lubrication tape, basin, and suction capability

(C) a contraindication to inserting the nasogastric tube is indigestion

(D) possible complications of nasogastric tube insertion include nasal trauma and insertion into the trachea

345. All of the following statements are true about performing the Sellick maneuver EXCEPT that

(A) this maneuver reduces gastric distention and prevents passive regurgitation

(B) to perform this maneuver, place your thumb and index finger on the sides of the midline on the cricoid ring

(C) after doing as described in B, exert firm pressure posteriorly, thus compressing the esophagus between the cricoid ring and the cervical spine without compromising the airway

(D) this maneuver can be started and discontinued several times during resuscitation, at 5- to 10-minute intervals

346. All of the following are indications for endotracheal intubation in the prehospital setting EXCEPT

(A) inability to ventilate an apneic patient

(B) a patient who is unresponsive to painful stimuli

(C) a patient who has a gag reflex

(D) a patient who cannot protect the airway (e.g., a patient in cardiac arrest)

347. Which of the following lists consists of equipment needed to properly perform endotracheal intubation?

(A) an endotracheal tube and a metal stylet

(B) a laryngoscope, a 10-cc syringe, and lubrication packets

(C) an oropharyngeal airway and tape

(D) a towel and a suction unit

348. All of the following statements regarding the curved laryngoscope blade and its use for endotracheal intubation are true EXCEPT that

(A) another name for the curved laryngoscope blade is the Apple blade

(B) it is used for adults only

(C) before using the curved laryngoscope blade, you must make sure that, when it locks into a perpendicular position, the light turns on

(D) before using the curved laryngoscope blade, you must make sure the light is bright and steady and that the bulb is tightly screwed in place

349. All of the following statements concerning the use of the straight laryngoscope blade, also known as the Miller blade, for endotracheal intubation are true EXCEPT that

(A) it is used for infants and children only

(B) before using the straight laryngoscope blade, you must make sure that, when it locks into a perpendicular position, the light turns on

(C) before using the straight laryngoscope blade, you must make sure that the light is bright and steady and that the bulb is tightly screwed in place

(D) the purpose of both the curved and the straight laryngoscope blades is to lift the epiglottitis out of the way to permit visualization of the airway

350. Which of the following is a true statement concerning the use of the stylet during endotracheal intubation?

(A) The stylet is inserted into the mouth in order to measure the distance of insertion of the endotracheal tube

(B) The stylet is held in the left hand, while the endotracheal tube is inserted with the right hand

(C) The stylet is inserted into the endotracheal tube to stiffen it

(D) The stylet is used to suction out the mouth after endotracheal intubation

351. All of the following statements about the proper size of endotracheal tubes for adults are true EXCEPT that

(A) the length of the adult endotracheal tube is 40 cm

(B) the size for an adult man is usually 8 to 8.5 mm

(C) the size for an adult woman is usually 7 to 8.0 mm

(D) in an emergency, a 7.5-mm tube will usually work for any adult

352. All of the following statements about the correct size of endotracheal tubes for infants and children are true EXCEPT that

(A) newborns and small infants need a 3- to 3.5-mm tube, and infants up to age 1 need a 4.0-mm tube

(B) charts and tape devices are usually inaccurate as a guide to selecting the right tube size

(C) the formula for selecting is (16 + age in years)/4

(D) the size of the child's fifth finger and the inside diameter of the nostril are both good indications of the correct tube size

353. All of the following are correct steps in preparing to perform endotracheal intubation in an adult EXCEPT

(A) administering 100% oxygen

(B) in a trauma patient, tilting the head, lifting the chin, and putting a towel under the head

(C) hyperventilating the patient at 24 breaths per minute for at least 2 minutes before intubation

(D) in a nontrauma patient, tilting the head, lifting the chin, and putting a towel under the head

354. All of the following are correct statements about the technique of performing endotracheal intubation in adults EXCEPT that

(A) with the laryngoscope in your left hand, you should lift the tongue and visualize the glottic opening and the vocal cords

(B) in lifting the laryngoscope blade, you must be careful to avoid putting pressure on the tongue

(C) with the right hand, you insert the endotracheal tube through the glottic opening until the cuff passes the vocal cords

(D) after you have inserted the endotracheal tube, you must remove the stylet

355. In preparing to perform endotracheal intubation in the infant or child, all of the following are true statements EXCEPT that

(A) you should administer 100% oxygen

(B) you should hyperventilate the patient at an age-appropriate rate

(C) if trauma is suspected, your partner should hold the patient's head in a neutral position

(D) if the patient has not suffered trauma, you should tilt the patient's head and lift the chin; infants may require a towel under the head to raise it about 5.0 cm

356. In performing endotracheal intubation in infants and children, all of the following are true EXCEPT that

(A) with the laryngoscope in your left hand, you should lift the tongue and visualize the glottic opening and the vocal cords

(B) in infants and children, tachycardia is a sign of oxygen deprivation

(C) you should lift the laryngoscope up and away from the patient, taking care to avoid pressure on the teeth

(D) after successful insertion of the endotracheal tube, you should remove the stylet

357. In the infant, child, and adult, the initial approach to confirming endotracheal tube placement is to listen for breath sounds over the apices and bases of both lungs and for the absence of gurgling sounds over the epigastrium. Other signs of correct endotracheal tube placement include all of the following EXCEPT

(A) improvement in the patient's heart rate, skin color, and general condition

(B) equal rise and fall of the chest during ventilation

(C) normal findings on pulse oximetry

(D) a decrease in mental status

358. Which of the following is the most dangerous complication of endotracheal intubation?

   (A) Damage to several teeth

   (B) Esophageal intubation

   (C) Placement of the endotracheal tube in a mainstem bronchus

   (D) Vomiting

359. All of the following are skills used in securing the properly placed endotracheal tube EXCEPT:

   (A) use of tape or a commercially available device

   (B) assessment of endotracheal tube placement by repeatedly trying to move the tube in and out of the patient's mouth

   (C) prevention of tube movement by manually holding the tube in place at the patient's mouth

   (D) frequent reevaluation of the tube placement, even after the tube has been secured

ADVANCED AIRWAY

A N S W E R S

339. The answer is C. [Mosby, Advanced Airway (Optional)] Compared to adults (*right*) children (*left*) have a tongue that is larger relative to the mouth, a glottis that is located more superiorly, and a cricoid area that is narrower.

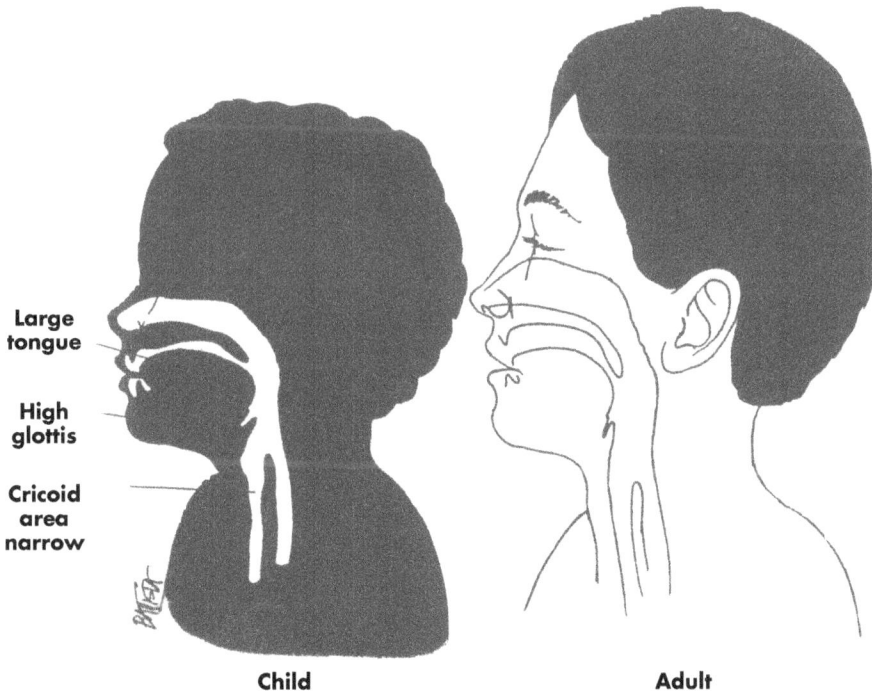

Large tongue

High glottis

Cricoid area narrow

Child   Adult

340. The answer is C. [Mosby, Advanced Airway (Optional)] The head is larger relative to the body in infants and children than in adults, and more of the skull projects posterior to the neck. Therefore, when an infant or child lies flat on the back, the head is forced into a flexed position, which can block the airway.

341. The answer is A. [Mosby, Advanced Airway (Optional)] In the unconscious adult, only artificial teeth (dentures or bridges) can slip back to obstruct the airway.

342. The answer is B. [Mosby, Advanced Airway (Optional)] An oropharyngeal airway cannot be inserted into any patient with a positive gag reflex. Doing so may cause gagging or vomiting, which can compromise the airway.

343. The answer is D. [Mosby, Advanced Airway (Optional)] The nonrebreather mask should fit from the bridge of the nose to just below the bottom lip.

344. The answer is C. [Mosby, Advanced Airway (Optional)] Indigestion is not a contraindication to insertion of the nasogastric tube. Instead, contraindications are major facial, head, or spinal trauma.

345. The answer is D. [Mosby, Advanced Airway (Optional)] Once you initiate the Sellick maneuver, it is important to maintain continuous pressure until the airway is protected with an endotracheal tube. Patients frequently vomit after cricoid pressure is released.

346. The answer is C. [Mosby, Advanced Airway (Optional)] One indication for endotracheal intubation is a patient who does NOT have a gag reflex. (The other indications are as given in choices A, B, and D.)

347. The answer is C. [Mosby, Advanced Airway (Optional)] An oropharyngeal (OP) airway or a bite block, with tape, is needed to prevent the patient from biting the endotracheal tube upon becoming responsive. A nasopharyngeal airway would not prevent this occurrence.

348. The answer is A. [Mosby, Advanced Airway (Optional)] Another name for the curved blade is the MacIntosh blade (not the "Apple" blade).

349. The answer is A. [Mosby, Advanced Airway (Optional)] This blade is used for adults as well as for infants and children.

350. The answer is C. [Mosby, Advanced Airway (Optional)] The stylet is a malleable piece of metal that is used to make the endotracheal tube stiff. This facilitates the insertion of the endotracheal tube.

351. The answer is A. [Mosby, Advanced Airway (Optional)] The length of the adult endotracheal tube is 33 cm.

352. **The answer is B.** [Mosby, Advanced Airway (Optional)] Charts and tapes are very helpful in indicating the correct size of the endotracheal tube to be used. The Braslow tape measures the child from head to toe and then calculates the correct size tube.

353. **The answer is B.** [Mosby, Advanced Airway (Optional)] In a trauma patient, your partner should stabilize the patient's head in a neutral position; the manipulations listed in B risk exacerbating or causing spinal cord injury.

354. **The answer is B.** [Mosby, Advanced Airway (Optional)] In lifting the laryngoscope blade, you must be careful to avoid putting pressure on the teeth.

355. **The answer is D.** [Mosby, Advanced Airway (Optional)] If infants require a towel, it should be placed under the upper back to raise the shoulders about 2.5 cm.

356. **The answer is B.** [Mosby, Advanced Airway (Optional)] In infants and children, bradycardia, not tachycardia, is a sign of oxygen deprivation.

357. **The answer is D.** [Mosby, Advanced Airway (Optional)] Correct endotracheal tube placement will not worsen mental status and may lead to improvement in it. Other means of checking for correct endotracheal tube placement are carbon dioxide detectors and tube-check devices.

358. **The answer is B.** [Mosby, Advanced Airway (Optional)] Misplacement of the tube into the esophagus is the most serious of the complications listed because it will prevent any oxygen from reaching the lungs. The patient will die unless the tube is immediately removed. Additional complications of endotracheal intubation are soft tissue trauma, decreased heart rate, hypoxia, and self-extubation.

359. **The answer is B.** [Mosby, Advanced Airway (Optional)] After the tube is secured, it should not be moved in or out of the patient's mouth. Tube placement should be reassessed any time the patient's condition changes.

BIBLIOGRAPHY

Crosby LA, Lewallen DG (eds.): *Emergency Care and Transportation of the Sick and Injured, 6/e*. Chicago, American Academy of Orthopedic Surgeons (AAOS), 1995.

Grant HD, Murray RH Jr., Bergeron JD, et al.: *Emergency Care*, 7/e. Boston, Brady, 1995.

Stoy WA (ed.): *Mosby's EMT-Basic Textbook*. St. Louis, Mosby-Lifeline, 1996.

www.ingramcontent.com/pod-product-compliance
Lightning Source LLC
Chambersburg PA
CBHW080559220326
41599CB00032B/6538